# Cognitive Remediation to Improve Functional Outcomes

# Cognitive Remediation to Improve Functional Outcomes

**EDITED BY**

**ALICE MEDALIA**

AND

**CHRISTOPHER R. BOWIE**

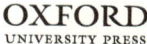

OXFORD
UNIVERSITY PRESS

# OXFORD
UNIVERSITY PRESS

Oxford University Press is a department of the University of Oxford. It furthers
the University's objective of excellence in research, scholarship, and education
by publishing worldwide.Oxford is a registered trade mark of Oxford University
Press in the UK and certain other countries.

Published in the United States of America by Oxford University Press
198 Madison Avenue, New York, NY 10016, United States of America.

Library of Congress Cataloging-in-Publication Data
Names: Medalia, Alice, editor. | Bowie, Christopher R., editor.
Title: Cognitive remediation to improve functional outcomes / edited by Alice
Medalia, Christopher R. Bowie.
Description: Oxford ; New York : Oxford University Press, [2016]
Identifiers: LCCN 2015036628 | ISBN 9780199395224 (paperback)
Subjects: LCSH: Cognition disorders—Patients—Rehabilitation. | Cognitive
therapy. | BISAC: PSYCHOLOGY / Clinical Psychology.
Classification: LCC RC553.C64 C662 2016 | DDC 616.89/1425—dc23 LC record available at http://lccn.
loc.gov/2015036628

9 8 7 6 5 4 3 2

Printed by Webcom, Canada

# CONTENTS

# ACKNOWLEDGMENTS

This book evolved from efforts that my co-editor, Alice Medalia, initiated years ago in an attempt to revolutionize how cognitive remediation effects can translate to improved everyday life for people dealing with mental illness. I am grateful for the opportunity to work with Alice to bring together an extraordinary team of the top clinician-scholars in our field who took the time to contribute to this volume with a thoughtful clinical tone that stayed rooted in empirical evidence. The cognitive remediation work we produce in my own laboratory comes from the opportunity to work with an exceptional research team at Queen's University including Maya Gupta, Katherine Holshausen, Michael Best, Michael Grossman, and Emma Ayukawa. It is important also to recognize the contributions of all of the individuals with mental illness who participate in the research process. I hope that the clinicians who use this book will find in it new ways to help improve the lives of those living with these conditions.

—Christopher Bowie, PhD

It has been a tremendous pleasure to work with my co-editor Christopher Bowie and the chapter authors who worked so carefully to inform clinical care with relevant research. I am grateful to the many Kessel and Stern Fellows who since 1996 have played an integral role in my laboratory, developing training methodologies that transfer cognitive skills to everyday functioning. I would also like to thank Connie and Steve Lieber for their support of the Lieber Recovery Clinic, a place where cognitive remediation is constantly being refined and perfected with invaluable input from patients, families, and clinicians. Finally, I would like to acknowledge those administrators of mental health care systems who have supported cognitive remediation initiatives. The feedback from clinicians and patients in these treatment settings has shaped the trajectory of cognitive remediation as it moves from research laboratory to clinical practice.

—Alice Medalia, PhD

## ABOUT THE EDITORS

**Alice Medalia, PhD,** is a Professor at Columbia University and an international leader in the field of psychiatric rehabilitation who is best known for her work in treating cognitive deficits in people with psychiatric disorders. Dr. Medalia has been instrumental in raising awareness about the need to address cognition as a central aspect of health related to functional outcome. She is the recipient of prestigious awards, a funded researcher, and a prolific author.

**Christopher Bowie, PhD,** is a clinical psychologist and Professor at Queen's University in Kingston, Ontario, and an Independent Scientist at the Centre for Addiction and Mental Health in Toronto, Ontario. His laboratory and clinical work focuses on the treatment of cognitive disorders in people with mental illness. He has developed new methods to enhance functioning through cognitive remediation techniques and has received several international recognitions for his research and practice.

**Christopher R. Bowie, PhD,** *Associate Professor of Psychology and Psychiatry; Director*, Cognitive and Psychotic Disorders Laboratory, Queen's University, Kingston, Ontario, Canada

**Adam Crowther, MSc,** *Research Worker*, Psychology Department, Institute of Psychiatry, Psychology and Neuroscience, King's College London, London, UK

**Frances Dark, PhD, MBBS, FRANZCP,** *Director*, Rehabilitation Academic Clinical Unit, Metro South Mental Health, Metro South Health Service, Brisbane, Australia

**Maya Gupta, MSc,** *Research Worker*, Cognitive and Psychotic Disorders Laboratory, Queen's University, Kingston, Ontario, Canada

**Philip D. Harvey, PhD,** *Leonard M. Miller Professor of Psychiatry and Behavioral Sciences; Chief of the Division of Psychology,* University of Miami Miller School of Medicine, Miami, Florida, USA

**Tiffany Herlands, PsyD,** *Assistant Professor of Medical Psychology*, Columbia University Medical Center; *Clinical Director*, Lieber Recovery and Rehabilitation Clinic, Columbia University Medical Center, New York, USA

**Katherine Holshausen, MSc,** *Research Worker*, Cognitive and Psychotic Disorders Laboratory, Queen's University, Kingston, Ontario, Canada

**William P. Horan, PhD,** *Associate Research Psychologist*, Department of Psychiatry & Biobehavioral Sciences, University of California Los Angeles, Los Angeles, California, USA

**Brett D. Jones, PhD,** *Professor,* Department of Learning Sciences & Technologies, Educational Psychology Program, Virginia Tech, Blacksburg, Virginia, USA

**Richard S. E. Keefe, PhD,** *Professor; Director*, Schizophrenia Research Group, Psychiatry & Behavioral Sciences, Division of Medical Psychology, School of Medicine, Duke University Medical Center, Durham, North Carolina, USA

**Matthew M. Kurtz, PhD,** *Associate Professor of Psychology and Neuroscience and Behavior,* Wesleyan University, Middletown, Connecticut; *Associate Professor (Adjunct) of Psychiatry,* Yale School of Medicine, New Haven, Connecticut, USA

**Alice Medalia, PhD,** *Clinical Director,* NY State OMH Cognitive Health Services; *Professor of Medical Psychology,* Columbia University Medical Center; *Director of Psychiatric Rehabilitation Services,* Columbia University College of Physicians and Surgeons, New York, USA

**Clare Reeder, PhD,** *Clinical Lecturer,* Psychology Department, Institute of Psychiatry, Psychology and Neuroscience, King's College London, London, UK

**David L. Roberts, PhD,** *Clinical Director,* Transitional Care Clinic, University of Texas Health Science Center at San Antonio, Psychiatry, San Antonio, Texas, USA

**Alice Saperstein, PhD,** *Assistant Professor of Medical Psychology,* Columbia University Medical Center, Columbia University College of Physicians & Surgeons, New York, USA

**Elizabeth W. Twamley, PhD,** Department of Psychiatry, University of California, San Diego; Center of Excellence for Stress and Mental Health, VA San Diego Healthcare System, San Diego, California, USA

**Til Wykes, PhD,** *Professor of Clinical Psychology and Rehabilitation; Vice Dean Psychology and Systems Science Psychology Department,* Institute of Psychiatry, Psychology and Neuroscience, King's College London, London, UK

Cognitive health is increasingly recognized as an important focus of mental health, because many psychiatric illnesses affect cognition, and the resulting deficits make it difficult to function independently in the community and engage in productive life activities. Psychiatric disorders are associated with abnormalities of affect, behavior, perception, and cognition. People can become depressed, psychotic, anxious, manic—but they also can have problems with memory, processing speed, and attention. For people to function effectively, they need emotional, physical, and cognitive health. They need to feel emotionally balanced, but they also need to be able to think clearly to negotiate daily tasks. We are most helpful to our patients when we address all their symptoms—including the cognitive ones.

Knowing that cognitive dysfunction is so prevalent among people with psychiatric diagnoses means that we need to carefully consider when and how to address cognitive problems. Both the "when" and the "how" questions involve the pivotal issue of the relevance of cognitive dysfunction to the ability of an individual to function in the community. Cognitive treatments are needed only if issues with cognition are hampering functioning, and the approach to treatment is most meaningful if it is personalized to address each person's goals for functioning in the community.

This book brings together the thinking of leading experts on treating cognition in the psychiatric disorders. In their individual chapters, these experts address the various ways in which cognitive treatments can be made relevant to functional outcome. Together, they emphasize the importance of putting cognitive treatments in a broader treatment context: to enhance daily functioning by building cognitive skills and the motivation to function in all aspects of life with maximum independence and success.

This broader treatment context is consistent with a recovery orientation. In recovery approaches, all treatment stems from a collaborative identification of clients' broader life goals and impediments to reaching those goals. Often this is easily accomplished, as when a patient who wants to return to school or work seeks treatment for the attention and memory problems that caused difficulty in those settings in the past. But just as often there is a less direct link between cognitive treatments and clients' identified goals. Perhaps, when asked what their goal was, the answer suggested an unrealistic appraisal of strengths and obstacles. This situation calls for a more nuanced therapeutic approach that emphasizes the role of individual clients' values and psychological needs in setting goals. Collaborative treatment planning can then proceed by listening carefully to what clients value (e.g., being a good worker, friend, child or parent; being smart; having social status), their psychological needs (e.g., to be successful, to feel in control, to have supportive people in their life), and their social system needs (e.g., housing, educational and economic opportunity). Cognitive remediation that proceeds from a base of careful listening and collaborative goal setting is more likely to have a positive impact, not just on cognition but on functioning in the community.

In this book, the various ways in which cognitive treatments can be refined to address functional goals are considered. The contributions of multiple experts on this topic provide perspectives not offered in other treatment manuals and books on cognitive remediation techniques. Readers will benefit from some basic skill acquisition, but ultimately the purpose is for active clinicians to refine their skill sets so that they can conduct cognitive enhancing treatments in a manner that increases the chances that cognitive gains will translate to improved quality of life and reduced disability. This book is thus intended to help the clinician take cognitive remediation from efficacy (improving cognition) to effectiveness (changing behavioral outcomes).

We start with a review of the evidence base for providing cognitive remediation and then proceed to the more procedural issues of performing an assessment and conducting sessions. One chapter is devoted to the systems issues—that is, the broader mental health systems context—that affect the delivery of cognitive remediation as a recovery-based treatment. Throughout this volume, the picture emerges that cognitive treatment can be grounded in both neuroscience and psychology, that it is both neuroplasticity and recovery based, and that it embraces both the proximal target of cognitive enhancement and the broader goal of improved community functioning.

Cognitive remediation for psychiatric populations has been developing as a therapy for more than 35 years. The proliferation of research and clinical interest invigorates the practice and strengthens its purpose, which ultimately is to improve the daily lives of people with mental illnesses. This book aims to provide a platform for further refinements of the practice of cognitive remediation. The message is that there is no one way to help improve cognition; rather, there are many ways, and the clinical challenge is to find what is right for the individual patient.

# Cognitive Remediation to Improve Functional Outcomes

# Cognitive Remediation for Psychological Disorders

## An Overview

**MATTHEW M. KURTZ** ∎

## INTRODUCTION

The clinician treating people with psychiatric illnesses—whether based at a community mental health center, in private practice, in a University medical setting, or at a long-term state inpatient unit—is confronted with an increasingly dizzying array of clinical manuals and off-the-shelf computerized exercises for improving thinking skills and associated functioning in people with psychiatric illnesses. The clinician may ask: What are the major programs of training in thinking skills from which to choose? Is there evidence that these programs work and will translate into functional improvements? How much training will I or my staff require to administer an intervention? What type of training in thinking skills is most appropriate for the type and mix of clients I treat? Will the effects of treatment on function last after treatment stops? How will different types of thinking skills training interact with other services offered by my agency, hospital, or private practice for improving functioning?

Interventions designed to improve thinking or cognitive skills are referred to as *cognitive remediation* (CR). CR has been defined as "a behavioral training based intervention that aims to improve cognitive processes (attention, memory, executive function, social cognition or meta-cognition) with the goal of durability and generalization" (Cognitive Remediation Experts Workshop, 2010, quoted in Barlati, Deste, De Peri, Ariu, & Vita, 2013). The first goal of this chapter is to provide an overall look at whistle-stop the three major types of CR that have emerged over the last 20 years—the compensatory/strategy-based, restorative, and social cognitive approaches. For each type, the theoretical rationale for the approach, its most common practice elements, and how the effects translate into changes in functioning are reviewed. Later chapters in this book provide detailed discussion of specific programmatic approaches for CR administration. Here, the focus is on the conceptual basis for doing CR, the research on efficacy and effectiveness of CR for psychiatric conditions, the nature of training for front-line clinicians administering the program, and what we know about the interaction of each class of intervention with other psychosocial rehabilitation interventions.

The second aim of this chapter is to help the clinician identify features of CR interventions and characteristics of the clients they serve that might help them make decisions about which CR approach will be most appropriate and who will benefit functionally. This section discusses the science of treatment response, what we know about who responds to which CR treatments, and how this information might be used to guide a thoughtful matching of CR interventions with the setting in which a clinician works and the mix of clients being treated.

The third aim of the chapter is to present two case studies of clients with psychiatric illness in a clinical setting. The deficits in thinking skills and other common features of the client's psychiatric disorder, the type of CR intervention administered, the progress of the client in treatment, and how improvements in CR skills were integrated into other domains of the client's life are discussed.

Because most clinical experience and research findings have been focused on people with schizophrenia, the largest emphasis in this chapter is placed on what we know regarding the application of CR for this psychiatric disorder. A section toward the end of the chapter details emerging clinical and research findings on the application of CR for other common psychiatric conditions, including mood disorders, attention-deficit hyperactivity disorder (ADHD), and hoarding disorder.

## RATIONALE FOR TREATMENT OF COGNITIVE DEFICITS

Among the first questions a clinician may ask, or may need to know to convince policymakers to fund programs of CR, is why is it important to treat deficits in thinking skills. There are two answers to this question. First, it is firmly established that cognitive deficits are a pervasive feature of many psychiatric disorders. For example, studies have shown that at least 70% of people with schizophrenia have cognitive profiles that would be rated as impaired by a clinical neuropsychologist (Palmer et al., 1997). Furthermore, when levels of cognitive capacity before disease onset are accounted for, all people with schizophrenia have some degree of cognitive impairment (Kurtz, Donato, & Rose, 2011; Wilk et al., 2005). This is in contrast to the frequency of several putatively characteristic psychiatric symptoms of schizophrenia that are used to inform diagnosis. Indeed, longitudinal studies have shown that two of the key symptoms long thought to be part of the core pathology of schizophrenia—delusions of control and auditory hallucinations commenting on one's behavior—are evident only in a subgroup of people with schizophrenia, even with a 20-year follow-up period (Rosen, Grossman, Harrow, Bonner-Jackson, & Faull, 2011). Therefore, cognitive deficits are more prevalent than key psychiatric symptoms of schizophrenia.

The second reason why it is important to treat deficits in thinking skills is that these deficits are moderately related to a broad array of measures of outcome. It is well established that cognitive deficits correlate with ratings of community function in which a client and, ideally, an informant are asked about the client's vocational status, number of friends, relationship with family, and participation in community activities such as attending concerts or borrowing books from the library (e.g., Green, Kern, Braff, & Mintz, 2000; Green, Kern & Heaton, 2004). Importantly, this relationship is evident both when cognitive deficits and community function are measured cross-sectionally (at the same time) and when these cognitive measures are used as predictors of subsequent outcome. Moreover, it holds both for clients with schizophrenia and for those with bipolar illness (e.g., Dickerson et al., 2010). Indeed, when compared directly, cognitive deficits play a larger role than severity of clinical symptoms in psychosocial outcomes of clients with schizophrenia.

Of equal concern to the clinician, cognitive deficits play a predominant role in the capacity of clients with schizophrenia to benefit from existing, evidence-based psychosocial rehabilitation interventions. For example, deficits in both attention and memory have been shown to affect the clinical response of patients with schizophrenia to evidence-based social skills treatment programs that are a mainstay of the rehabilitation armamentarium (Kern, Green, & Satz, 1992; Mueser, Bellack, Douglas, & Wade, 1991). First, these deficits appear to interfere with the acquisition of elementary social skills, such as enhanced eye contact, improved voice tone and volume, and goal-directed communications, that are crucial for translating treatment effects into improved functioning in the community. Second, those clients with greater cognitive deficits are less likely to attend treatment sessions (McKee, Hull, & Smith, 1997). In work therapy programs also, summary measures of cognition and executive function, along with thought disorder, influence assessments of on-the-job work skills in supervised settings (Bell & Bryson, 2001; Lysaker, Bell, Zito, & Bioty, 1995). Other studies have shown that executive function, along with negative symptoms, influence real-world, competitive job outcomes as measured by hours worked and wages earned (McGurk & Mueser, 2006; McGurk, Mueser, Harvey, LaPuglia, & Marder, 2003). Finally, cognitive deficits also play a role in more integrated programs of rehabilitation that include many treatment elements such as social skills training, psychoeducation, treatment of substance abuse, vocational counseling, and motivation groups. Here, too, higher scores on measures of cognition, specifically attention and verbal and nonverbal memory, all predicted a better response to integrated psychosocial treatment (e.g., Brekke, Hoe, Long, & Green, 2007; Kurtz, Wexler, Fujimoto, Shagan, & Seltzer, 2008). These results have been consistent across studies, with both inpatients and outpatients.

Taken together, these findings suggest that cognitive deficits, which are almost universally present in people with a diagnosis of schizophrenia, play a foundational role in functional status and rehabilitation treatment response, both in clients in acute states and in those that are stabilized as outpatients, and therefore must be a central treatment target of any structured program of rehabilitation.

## METHODS OF COGNITIVE REMEDIATION

For the purposes of this chapter, CR approaches can be divided into three major intervention categories. *Strategy-based/compensatory approaches* focus on acquiring skills or modifying the environment to circumvent cognitive difficulties. In some cases, the therapist provides cognitive supports for a contextually placed, ecologically relevant task at first (e.g., planning a trip to the beach), reviews these supports with the client, and then allows the client to practice cognitive strategies as the therapist gradually removes the supports. In other cases, the client's home environment is modified directly, for example by placing signs and equipment in front of the client at a key home location to provide cueing and sequencing for the completion of an everyday life task (e.g., teeth brushing).

*Restorative approaches* target cognitive deficits directly through repeated task practice, careful titration of task difficulty, and maintenance of high levels of accurate performance. This approach can be likened to that of a physical therapist who prescribes consistent and sustained exercise for muscle groups that have atrophied due to disuse or structural damage. In these interventions, task practice is typically organized hierarchically, with elementary aspects of sensory processing or attention trained first, followed by training in higher-order memory and problem-solving skills. These approaches often rest on the assumption that improvements in cognition are mediated by neuroplasticity and lead to more accurate sensory representations of environmental stimuli, thereby enhancing the output of computational cognitive systems. Importantly, these approaches are not mutually exclusive from strategy approaches. Indeed, cognitive strategies such as combining individual items of information into larger meaningful groups based on shared stimulus characteristics for enhanced recall can be added to restorative exercises, and this is usually done by a therapist, although recently some computer exercises have been designed to include strategy coaching.

*Social cognitive approaches* focus on ameliorating deficits in taking others' perspectives (theory of mind), recognizing expressed affect, and retraining information processing biases (e.g., attention to threat-related information), which are hypothesized to produce delusional thought processes. They apply principles of repetition, modeling, role-playing, and corrective feedback to enhance social cognitive skills.

## Strategy-Based/Compensatory Training

Strategy-based and compensatory remediation interventions rely on several key principles: (1) teaching new, efficient, information processing strategies; (2) aiding the transfer of cognitive gains to the real world; and (3) modifying the local environment of the client to enhance the likelihood of successful completion of everyday life activities. Program modules may target specific cognitive skills such as cognitive flexibility, memory, and planning, using cognitive exercises that are graded in difficulty to minimize task-related errors and promote errorless learning. Often, the exercises are contextualized in real-world activities such as organizing a bus trip from one's hometown to the town of a friend for a lunch date. In some cases, clinicians visit a client's home and modify the living environment directly.

## Restorative Training

Restorative CR interventions are usually computer assisted and present hierarchically organized programs in which simpler neurocognitive functions are trained before more complex functions. They rely heavily on task practice and carefully titrate task difficulty according to the individual participant's ability level. The primary hypothesis of the approach is that minimizing invocation of verbally mediated guidance and other superordinate executive cognitive mechanisms, and instead placing emphasis on implicit practice-related learning, will facilitate acquisition of elementary cognitive skills in schizophrenia. A corollary assumption is that any evident improvements in elementary cognition will generalize to other key features of the disorder. Exercises typically begin at the individually determined level of difficulty at which the client is successful (e.g., 80% accuracy); this presumably helps engage underfunctioning brain systems and maintain high levels of positive reinforcement. An example of the type of exercise used in this program is presented in Figure 1.1.

Restorative programs vary in the degree to which they emphasize the most basic cognitive skills (e.g., sensory processing). Some programs start by improving the speed and accuracy of auditory information processing, whereas others start with basic attention. Ongoing research seeks to understand the best way to use these approaches in clinical practice; to date, benefits to cognition have been shown with restorative programs that emphasize a range of cognitive skills. For example, restorative programs targeting elementary sensory processing have produced substantial improvements in verbal learning and memory that persist for at least 6 months (Fisher, Holland, Merzenich, & Vinogradov, 2009; Fisher, Holland, Subramanian, & Vinogradov, 2010), whereas those targeting sustained attention, memory, executive function, and language have produced improvements in working memory, problem solving, and facial affect recognition (Bell, Bryson, Greig, Corcoran, & Wexler, 2001).

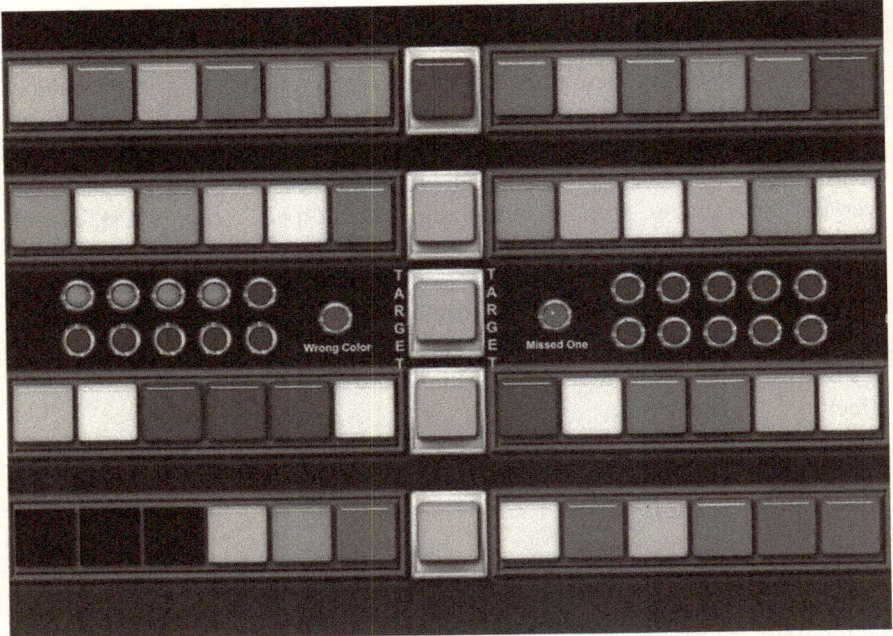

**Figure 1.1** Screenshot from the task "Simultaneous Multiple Attention" by Odie Bracy, PhD. This is a prototypical example of a restorative, drill-and-practice exercise that includes the ability to carefully titrate task difficulty. It represents an intermediate stage (shifting attention) in a hierarchically ordered program of cognitive remediation exercises.
From Bracy, O. (1995). *PSS CogRehab,* version 95. Psychological Software Services, Inc., Indianapolis, IN.

## Social Cognitive Training

Although a range of initial proof-of-concept studies have provided evidence that two key domains of social cognition, facial affect recognition and theory of mind, can be improved with relatively brief interventions consisting of attentional prompts, verbalization strategies, and didactic instruction, only in the last 8 to 10 years have comprehensive, sustained, stand-alone treatments for multiple domains of social cognitive deficits been developed (Kurtz & Richardson, 2012). Comprehensive programs of social cognitive training are designed to address multiple impairments in social cognition in clients with schizophrenia (Horan et al., 2011; Penn, Roberts, Combs, & Sterne, 2007). They consist of modules typically administered in small groups of clients who meet weekly for several months. Unlike neurocognitive training, social cognitive training often uses video recordings and role-playing and targets both deficits and biases in information processing. Complex social cognitive processes are broken into component skills, which are taught using combinations of heuristic rehearsal, modeling, task practice, and role-playing with corrective feedback.

## IS COGNITIVE REMEDIATION
## AN EVIDENCE-BASED PRACTICE?

A common approach to determining whether a health care intervention constitutes an evidence-based practice is whether, when the results of all existing studies of the treatment are combined, there is evidence of meaningful improvement on outcomes targeted by the intervention (i.e., *proximal outcomes*). The intervention is regarded even more positively if its effects generalize to outcomes that might be related to the proximal outcome and might have broader clinical significance but are not directly targeted by the intervention itself (i.e., *distal measures*). In the case of CR, improvements on measures of cognition (e.g., attention, memory, problem solving), compared with study entry scores or with a control group tested over a similar time interval, are an indication of effectiveness on proximal measures, whereas improvements in symptoms, functioning, or relapse indicate generalization of cognitive training procedures to distal outcome measures. The issue of proximal versus distal treatment targets takes on particular salience in schizophrenia research because identification of a core pathology remains elusive and detailed models linking cognitive skills, function, and symptoms are lacking.

Quantitatively combining multiple studies into what has been labeled a *meta-analysis* is a commonly accepted, objective way of assessing the evidence base of a new treatment. The advantage of this approach, as opposed to literary reviews of the scholarly corpus, is that it permits a formal combination of results across studies. Findings from each study are placed on a common metric, called an *effect size*, which is measured by Cohen's $d$ (Cohen, 1997); this weights the studies by their respective sample sizes, after which the results are combined. Differences in characteristics of the studies that comprise the analysis (e.g., sample age, duration of illness, type of pharmacotherapy) can then be analyzed by what has been labeled meta-regression. In meta-analyses of CR studies, $d$-values represent the difference between the treatment condition (i.e., some type of cognitive training) and the control condition (e.g., treatment as usual, computer games, some alternative form of learning program) at the end of the CR intervention on a specific outcome measure. This difference is divided by the average variability on that same measure from one participant to another treated within the same group (treatment or control). As a benchmark, the following commonly accepted ranges are used to define the magnitude of effect sizes: small, $d = .2$ to $.4$; medium, $d = .4$ to $.8$; and large, $d > .8$ (Cohen, 1977).

Studies of CR have generated great interest from meta-analysts, and to date, nine meta-analyses or effect-size analyses have been conducted and reported in the peer-reviewed literature. Eight of these meta-analyses replicated one another and concluded that CR outperformed control conditions on proximal cognitive outcomes, with effect sizes ranging from small to large ($d = .3$ to almost 1.0) (Fig. 1.2). The large value from the paper by Kurtz, Moberg, Gur, and Gur (2001) is an outlier related to the fact that the analysis relied exclusively on studies using cognitive outcome measures that were identical

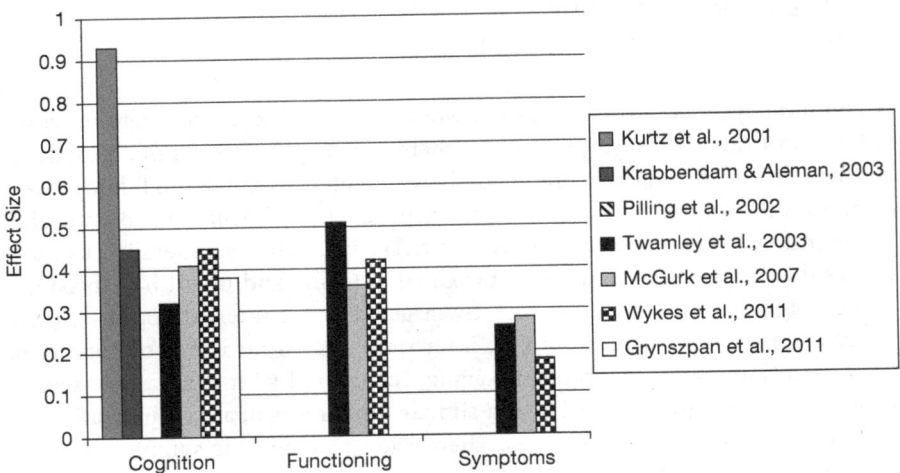

**Figure 1.2** Effects of cognitive remediation on cognition, function, and symptoms in schizophrenia: results from effect size and formal meta-analyses.
From Kurtz, M. M. (2015). Cognitive and social cognitive interventions for schizophrenia. In Nathan, P. & Gorman, J. (Eds.). *A guide to treatments that work* (4th ed.). New York: Oxford University Press. Reprinted by permission of Oxford University Press, USA www.oup.com.

to the cognitive domains trained in CR. Other values largely reflect effects of CR on cognitive outcomes that are not directly trained in the treatment. Therefore, CR clearly produces mild to moderate improvement in cognition, and in a subgroup of these studies ($n = 11$) it was shown that these effects are durable, lasting as long as 8 months (Wykes, Huddy, Cellard, McGurk, & Czobor, 2011). Moreover, the effects of these interventions under some circumstances generalize to functioning, with mean effect sizes in the small to moderate range ($d = .35$ to $.5$) and larger effects when CR is offered along with other rehabilitative interventions. The effects of CR on symptoms have typically been modest and frequently nonsignificant.

## DOES COGNITIVE REMEDIATION IMPROVE FUNCTIONING?

The balance of evidence to date suggests that CR programs improve functioning when offered with other rehabilitative interventions for people with schizophrenia. This claim is based on the effects of combined treatments in CR studies that embedded their treatment within other rehabilitative services such as structured social or work skills training, compared with the results from studies of stand-alone CR interventions offered without these psychosocial interventions. But, in creating a rationale for the addition of a new program of CR to existing clinical services, the clinical administrator may want to know whether there is specific evidence showing that CR provides a meaningful increase in the effectiveness of existing psychosocial treatments for producing change in functional outcome when compared with the same treatment provided without CR—and, if so, what is the status of the relative evidence of transfer of cognitive training effects to real-world outcomes in the three conceptual models discussed earlier in this chapter?

With respect to the first question, initial results are quite promising. In an important study, Bowie, McGurk, Mausbach, Patterson, and Harvey (2012) compared the effects of a hybrid program of restorative and strategy-based CR treatment and functional skills training on measures of targeted outcomes and more general measures of psychosocial function, both independently and when the two treatments were combined and administered sequentially. Results clearly revealed that CR administered alone produced cognitive gains but no effect on community function measures; skills training produced change in the functional skills taught but had little effect on community function measures; and the combined treatments offered sequentially produced greater effects on measures of community function than either treatment alone. Therefore, enhanced cognitive skills permitted clients in this study to take better advantage of functional skills training, possibly by enhanced acquisition of elementary functional skills in groups, which then transferred more effectively to ratings of real-world community function. Perhaps even more remarkably, positive results on competitive employment outcomes have been reported for the addition of CR programs to evidence-based supported employment interventions. In these studies, the addition of CR produced meaningful and substantial changes in real-world outcome measures that are among those most highly valued by both consumers and clinicians: hours worked and wages earned in competitively obtained employment (e.g., McGurk, Mueser, & Pascaris, 2005).

With respect to the second question, there is some evidence that incorporating strategy-focused instruction into the CR program produces improvement in ratings of actual functioning (Wykes et al., 2011). Restorative approaches used in isolation are shown to most consistently benefit cognition, with little change in functional outcome, but when they are combined with strategy approaches, both cognition and functioning are improved. Social cognitive training programs produce improvements in inpatient ward behavior and outpatient ratings of community function (Kurtz & Richardson, 2012). Therefore, empirical studies suggest that combining approaches is both feasible and beneficial for psychosocial function. Table 1.1 provides a summary of key research studies supporting the use of CR, typically along with other rehabilitative interventions, to improve functioning.

*Table 1.1.* SELECTED RESEARCH STUDIES SHOWING EFFECTS OF COGNITIVE REMEDIATION (CR) PSYCHOSOCIAL AND WORK FUNCTION IN PEOPLE WITH PSYCHOLOGICAL DISORDERS

| Study | Psychological Disorder | Inpatients or Outpatients | Type of CR Program | Treatment Setting | Other Psychosocial Interventions Offered | Effects on Function |
|---|---|---|---|---|---|---|
| SOCIAL AND COMMUNITY FUNCTION OUTCOMES | | | | | | |
| Bowie et al., 2012 | Chronic schizophrenia | Outpatients | Hybrid restorative and strategy-based CR with bridging groups | Academic outpatient clinics | Life skills training | Improved ratings of community function |
| Eack et al., 2009 | Early-stage schizophrenia | Outpatients | CET: Restorative cognitive training and social cognitive interventions | State psychiatric clinic, academically affiliated | None reported | Improved scores on measures of social adjustment |
| Hogarty et al., 2004 | Chronic schizophrenia | Outpatients | CET: Restorative cognitive training and social cognitive interventions | Academic outpatient clinic | None reported | Improved scores on measures of social adjustment and activities of daily living |
| Roberts et al., 2014 | Chronic schizophrenia | Outpatients | Social Cognitive Training Program (SCIT) | Community mental health centers | None reported | Improvement on ratings of social function and performance-based social function |

| | | | | | | |
|---|---|---|---|---|---|---|
| Spaulding et al., 1999 | Chronic schizophrenia | Inpatients | Cognitive subprogram of Integrated Psychological Therapy (IPT) | State psychiatric facility | Social and living skills training, behavior modification, occupational therapy, psychoeducaton, and family education | Improvement on a performance-based measure of skills for sending and receiving social information |
| Twamley et al., 2012 | Chronic primary psychotic disorder | Outpatients | Compensatory cognitive training | Community mental health centers | None specified | Improvement in performance-based measures of activities of daily living |
| WORK OUTCOMES | | | | | | |
| Bell et al., 2005 | Chronic schizophrenia or schizoaffective disorder | Outpatients | Restorative Training (Bracy exercises) and bridging groups | VA hospital | Work therapy programs | Hours worked and wages earned in VA-sponsored employment |
| Bell et al., 2008 | Chronic schizophrenia or schizoaffective disorder | Outpatients | Restorative Training (Bracy exercises and Scientific Learning) and bridging groups | Urban community mental health center | Hybrid supported employment and vocational rehabilitation program | Cumulative rates of competitive employment higher in individuals treated with CR and vocational services compared with vocational services alone over a 2-year period |

(continued)

Table 1.1. CONTINUED

| Study | Psychological Disorder | Inpatients or Outpatients | Type of CR Program | Treatment Setting | Other Psychosocial Interventions Offered | Effects on Function |
|-------|------------------------|---------------------------|--------------------|-------------------|------------------------------------------|---------------------|
| WORK OUTCOMES | | | | | | |
| Eack et al., 2011 | Early-stage schizophrenia | Outpatients | CET: Restorative cognitive training and social cognitive interventions | State psychiatric clinic, academically affiliated | None reported | Increased likelihood of employment, number of hours worked, and satisfaction with the job over the 2-year study period |
| Lindenmayer et al., 2008 | Schizophrenia, schizoaffective disorder, and bipolar disorder | Inpatients | Restorative training (Thinking Skills for Work Program) and bridging groups | State psychiatric facility | Vocational program | Increased number of weeks worked in hospital-sponsored employment |
| McGurk et al., 2005 | Schizophrenia, schizoaffective disorder, and mood disorder | Outpatients | Restorative training (Thinking Skills for Work Program) and bridging groups | Urban community mental health centers | Supported employment | Likelihood of working, number of jobs, hours worked, and wages earned in competitive employment over a 1-year period. |

NOTE: All studies represent randomized, controlled trials, and reported effects on function represent a statistically significant difference between a CR-treated group and a control group. CET = cognitive enhancement therapy; VA = Veterans Administration.

# WHAT PARTICIPANT FACTORS INCREASE THE LIKELIHOOD OF A POSITIVE RESPONSE TO COGNITIVE REMEDIATION?

Given the time- and cost-intensive nature of many of the CR programs described in this chapter, it is crucial that CR treatments be carefully matched to clients who possess features that suggest they are most likely to benefit. Likewise, those factors that predict a poor response to CR should be taken into account when designing the next generation of CR therapies to maximize their effects for the largest number of people with mental illness. Although the literature on participant factors that influence treatment response is sparse, some conclusions can be offered.

Among the first studies to investigate these issues was by Medalia and Richardson (2005). Using three databases, they applied their NEAR motivational CR approach (Medalia, Revheim, & Herlands, 2009) to mixed samples that included a majority of people with schizophrenia and schizoaffective disorder (about 30% of the sample had a mood disorder instead). Figure 1.3 shows an example of stimuli used to enhance motivational engagement in this approach. The authors selected a reliable change index as a statistical procedure to define improvement. This procedure is applied on an individual client level and indicates when the magnitude of improvement on a specific outcome measure could have occurred by chance fewer than 5 of 100 times, accounting for the test-retest instability associated with the particular measure under study. Using this approach, each client in a sample was classified as either an "improver" or a "nonimprover." The first key finding from the study was that the number of clients who improved in each sample ranged from 40% to 69% of the total sample from which they were culled, so there was clearly considerable heterogeneity in treatment response that demands explanation. The second key finding was that most of the illness and demographic factors studied in their report (e.g., age, education, socioeconomic status, pattern and severity of symptoms) had a minimal effect on reported outcomes. Only level of motivation (as indexed by frequency of attendance at groups) and work style factors rated by clinicians prior to study entry (e.g., social skill, cooperativeness, task focus) were key factors for predicting a good treatment response.

More recent studies have amplified these results. For example, Kurtz, Seltzer, Fujimoto, Shagan, and Wexler (2009), in a sample of people with chronic schizophrenia, found that elementary sustained attention and working memory, as measured by a digit span task, predicted those who were most likely to show improved functional outcome after an extensive (mean, 70 hours) restorative program of CR, even when other key cognitive variables were controlled. Fiszdon, Cardenas, Bryson, and Bell (2005), using another chronic schizophrenia sample and a drill-and-practice restorative program almost identical to that of Kurtz study, found that measures of hostility, duration of time between termination of training and follow-up, and scores on measures of attention and immediate memory predicted the likelihood that scores on an exercise that was an element of the CR program itself would be in the normal range. A subsequent study by the same group revealed that premorbid IQ levels had an impact on the generalization of training effects (Fiszdon, Choi, Bryson, & Bell, 2006).

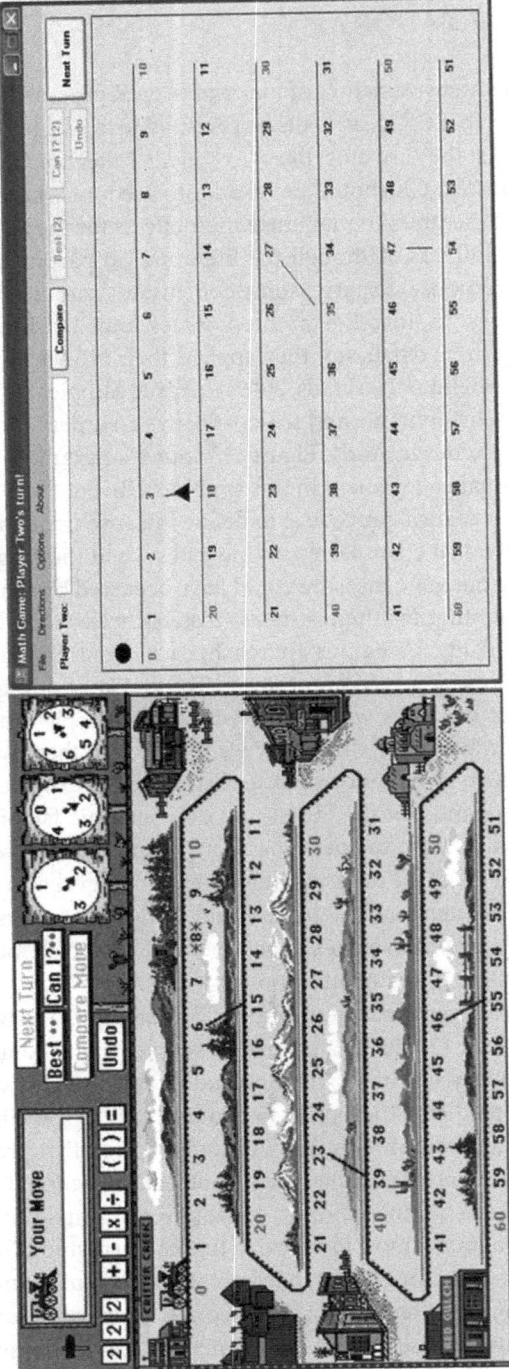

Figure 1.3 *Left panel*, Math game with multimodal stimulus features designed to increase intrinsic motivation in the participant. The approach includes personalization of the learning environment through choice in the selection of a game theme (in this case, "Critter Creek"). *Right panel*, Depiction of the same task without these motivational features. From Choi, J., & Medalia, A. (2010). Intrinsic motivation and learning in a schizophrenia-spectrum sample. *Schizophrenia Research 118*, 12–19. Reprinted with kind permission from Elsevier.

The role of participant age in CR treatment response has been studied in two reports (Kontis, Huddy, Reeder, Landau, & Wykes, 2013; Wykes et al., 2009). These studies evaluated the effects of a strategy-based form of CR called cognitive remediation therapy (i.e., CRT) in people with schizophrenia who were younger or older than 40 years of age and compared them with the results in a control group. Improvements were evident in planning and negative symptoms, relative to controls, only in the younger group. These findings were consistent even when measures of premorbid intellectual functioning were accounted for; higher estimated premorbid intellectual function predicted only the degree of practice effects evident on repeated administration of measures of working memory (regardless of age group assignment).

On the other hand, there was no indication of an effect of age on CR effect sizes in the meta-analysis done on 40 CRT trials (Wykes et al., 2011). Furthermore, age did not differentiate improvers from nonimprovers in the Medalia and Richardson's (2005) analysis of factors that predicted response to the NEAR method of CR. The impact of age on CR response is still being investigated, and factors that may interact with age, such as length of treatment and type of CR, are also being considered.

Expert opinion indicates that the following participant factors are associated with clients who are most likely to benefit from cognitive remediation and show improved functional outcomes:

1. High levels of client cooperativeness
2. Less-impaired skills in elementary attention and memory
3. Motivation for treatment success (as indexed by treatment attendance)
4. Estimated premorbid IQ >70 (at least Borderline Normal)

Surprisingly, other key psychiatric features, such as positive and negative symptoms in schizophrenia, have largely failed to show a relationship to treatment response and should not influence decisions on treatment application. Taken together, these factors suggest which clients are most likely to benefit, but CR still might be advantageous to others. In addition, several of the chapters in this volume outline approaches for addressing key factors on this list: improving motivation and cooperativeness for CR and enhancing elementary skills in attention and memory.

## WHAT CHARACTERISTICS OF THE INTERVENTION INCREASE THE LIKELIHOOD OF A POSITIVE RESPONSE TO COGNITIVE REMEDIATION?

The intervention characteristics that enhance the likelihood of a positive response to CR remain largely understudied; key intervention features such as treatment duration and intensity have yet to be manipulated directly as an independent variable in any study of CR. Meta-analyses to date (e.g., McGurk, Twamley, Sitzer, McHugo, & Mueser, 2007; Wykes et al., 2011) have not identified effects of treatment length on proximal or distal outcomes in CR studies despite wide ranges in the duration of training. For example, the studies analyzed by Wykes and colleagues ranged from 3 to 126 targeted hours of treatment and, in terms of intensity, from less than 1 hour per week to 5 hours of training per week. It is possible that effects of treatment duration could be obscured by the aggregation of results across very different treatment methodologies. Kurtz and colleagues (2009) used a drill-and-practice restorative approach and saw no effects of CR treatment duration or intensity on changes in functional capacity. Indeed, the only exception to these findings was reported by Choi and Medalia (2005) and Medalia and Richardson (2005), who showed that change did not occur on cognitive outcomes in their NEAR CR program when clients attended less than a threshold of two treatment sessions per week.

In the only study to evaluate the effects of the level of training of the therapist on CR outcomes, Medalia and Richardson (2005), using the motivational NEAR approach to CR (Medalia et al., 2009), found that NEAR groups involving a PhD-level therapist doing a postdoctoral fellowship in CR were more likely to produce improved cognitive function in their clients than groups led by therapists with Master's, Bachelor's, or Associate-level degrees who had little dedicated time for doing CR and little say in whether they were to run the groups. The authors hypothesized that the different client treatment outcomes reflected not only the level of training but also motivational and administrative support variables. They noted that the PhD-level staff in their sample had voluntarily made a commitment to learn about cognitive treatments, whereas the other clinicians were assigned by administrators to run the groups and may have had weaker identification with the role of a CR therapist and lower levels of motivation to address cognition.

One clear conclusion from most recent meta-analyses is that when programs of CR are paired with other psychosocial rehabilitative interventions, their effects are much more likely to generalize to more distal psychosocial function measures (Wykes et al., 2011). Indeed, effects of CR on measures of function are in the moderate range ($d = .59$) when paired with these interventions but in the small range ($d = .28$) and not statistically significant when CR is offered as a stand-alone treatment. Which conceptual models of CR can be most profitably integrated with which specific methods of evidence-based psychosocial interventions remains a key future question for the field.

Expert opinion suggests the following conclusions about which characteristics of CR interventions are most likely to produce positive functional outcomes:

1. For translation of CR effects to functional outcomes, CR must include explicit techniques for developing skills and must be paired with other evidence-based psychosocial treatments (e.g., supported employment programs, work therapy, functional or social skills training) or otherwise provided in the context of a recovery-oriented treatment program.
2. Clear recommendations regarding the optimal length of CR interventions remain unknown. Nonetheless, some broad guidelines can be offered. Positive effects have been shown in some cases with relatively brief CR interventions (approximately 3 months) and with CR interventions of lower intensity (as low as two times per week).

3. Therapists with graduate-level training concerning cognitive functioning in psychiatric patients, who seek out training in CR and are given dedicated time to learn about and do CR, are likely to be more effective in producing positive functional outcomes.

## SUMMARY OF COGNITIVE REMEDIATION IN SCHIZOPHRENIA AND RELATED PSYCHIATRIC DISORDERS

Impairments in attention, memory, problem-solving, and other cognitive skills in schizophrenia and related psychiatric disorders are almost universal, are resistant to the effects of optimal pharmacotherapy, impair community function, and interfere with the acquisition of key living skills in psychosocial rehabilitation. Over the last 20 years, several models of CR for improving cognitive function in people with psychiatric illness have been identified, including strategy-based, restorative, and social cognitive programs. Studies summarizing the results of 40 controlled trials using these methods have revealed small to moderate effects of CR on cognitive outcomes. Furthermore, effects of CR have been shown to generalize to measures of function when paired with other psychosocial interventions. Therefore, CR is an evidence-based practice that can serve as a key element of any rehabilitative armamentarium of treatments for schizophrenia.

To date, no clear evidence supports one CR treatment approach over another, so clinicians planning to implement CR in their clinical service need to consider the features of their client populations and unit resources (e.g., availability of computers, costs of purchasing software, level of training of relevant staff) as key factors in their decision-making process. Although data on client and treatment factors that promote a good response to CR remain scant and have been collected from studies using vastly different approaches to CR, cooperativeness, motivation, younger age, elementary attention and memory skills, and higher estimated premorbid IQ all suggest a better response to treatment. With respect to intervention factors, pairing of CR with other psychosocial interventions is the most powerful predictor of generalization of CR effects to functioning.

## EXPANSION OF COGNITIVE REMEDIATION ACROSS PSYCHIATRIC DIAGNOSES

Neuropsychological impairment has been identified as a core impairment in major depressive disorder (e.g., Porter, Gallagher, Thompson, & Young, 2003), bipolar illness during both acute episodes and periods of euthymia (Kurtz & Gerraty, 2009), ADHD (Van Hulst, de Zeeuw, & Durston, 2014), and hoarding disorder (Tolin, Villavicencio, Umbach, & Kurtz, 2011), among other psychiatric diagnoses. Although the links between observed deficits and functional impairment are less well established, the findings in clients with schizophrenia suggest that CR approaches could be of therapeutic value in these disorders as well. Pilot work has revealed improvements in attention deficits in people with treatment-resistant depression (Bowie et al., 2013), ADHD (Stevenson, Whitmont, Bornholt, Livesey, & Stevenson, 2002), and hoarding disorder (DiMauro, Genova, Tolin, & Kurtz, 2014) who were treated with forms of CR similar to those studied in schizophrenia. The expansion of CR treatment to other psychiatric disorders is an exciting development in the field, with many new randomized controlled trials ongoing.

## CASE EXAMPLES

### Effective Treatment with Cognitive Remediation in Schizophrenia

Jeffrey, a 23-year-old Caucasian male with a 3-year history of schizophrenia, was living at his parents' home with considerable financial and psychosocial support. He was diagnosed when he became convinced that the Central Intelligence Agency was sending him personal messages through newspaper articles in the *New York Times* about an upcoming invasion of the United States by Russia. His delusions became so prominent that he was forced to drop out of college during his sophomore year, at which time he moved back to his home of origin. Jeffrey then became isolative, spending most of his days alone in his childhood room in his parents' house. He used packing tape to keep all his windows and doors shut, and he covered each window with bedsheets. His hygiene and ability to carry out other activities of daily living declined markedly. As his symptoms worsened at home, he underwent a brief hospitalization at the psychiatric unit of a local hospital. Jeffrey was treated with a course of olanzapine, which was maintained on an ongoing basis through his local community mental health center after his discharge. Over a period of several weeks, medication produced a remarkable reduction in his delusions, although on occasion he stated that he had read an article in the paper that made him suspicious of an imminent invasion. He remained largely isolative but no longer felt the need to tape his windows and doors shut, and he engaged with his parents in conversation from time to time. With his greater psychiatric stability, Jeffrey was interested in restarting his college studies, but he encountered considerable difficulty concentrating and remembering things, and as a result, he and his parents were concerned about his ability to succeed. At the community mental health center, he was assessed with a brief neurocognitive test battery. Results revealed relatively strong sustained attention but mild to moderate difficulties in divided attention, working memory, verbal episodic memory, and spatial memory. He enrolled in a program which he attended 3 days per week, 1 hour per day, with five other clients. The program started with exercises targeted at simple sustained attention, from which Jeffrey graduated rapidly, achieving strong scores. He spent extended time on exercises targeted at his areas of specific difficulty, working on skills in divided attention before moving on to more complex, multicomponent cognitive skills such as working memory and verbal list learning. A bridging group was offered, and Jeffrey was able to discuss the impact of his cognitive deficits in his day-to-day life. A therapist worked with him individually on strengthening study skills and improving time management and note-taking and also provided psycho-education concerning the need for continued psychiatric medications. By the end of his 6 months of sustained CR treatment, Jeffrey's divided attention and working memory were within normal levels, and he enrolled in two community college courses, his first classes since leaving college 3 years before.

## Effective Treatment with Cognitive Remediation in Bipolar Illness

Judy, a 46-year-old, divorced mother of two with a 22-year history of bipolar illness with intermittent medication adherence, was living on disability insurance income in a private apartment with Section 8 housing support. Although she was estranged from her two adult daughters, Judy had a sister who provided financial and psychosocial support and visited on a regular basis. At the time of the start of CR treatment, Judy was spending much of her day at home, largely isolated from others. When her mood was stable enough, she devoted much of her time to creating origami sculptures in her apartment; she had taught origami in the public school system before her illness. Although she was still subject to episodes of persistent weeping and suicidal ideation, these episodes had become fewer and shorter over time. A brief assessment of neuro-cognitive skills on entry to her community mental health center revealed mild deficits in verbal learning and memory and executive function. An assessment identified her goal of obtaining a volunteer position at the local hospital to help with blood drives by providing support for donors to register at the entry desk. A 3-month, twice-a-week course of CR was offered with a focus on reducing impulsive responding. The CR therapist focused on providing scaffolding for cognitive tasks. The therapist initiated treatment by guiding information processing directly, for example by pointing to individual items on a cognitive training measure slowly and sequentially, as a strategy for slowing down Judy's rapid and often inaccurate response processing. As processing became less impulsive, these supports were gradually removed. Weekly cognitive processing discussion groups focused on how inhibiting rapid, emotionally driven stimulus-response reactions can reduce negative interactions with others in the work setting. Slowing down thoughts and actions and considering alternative interpretations and responses became a focus of discussion for several weeks. Judy's attendance at treatment groups improved during the 3-month intervention; her adherence to prescribed medication improved, and she began work in her chosen volunteer profession.

## Conclusion

Both of these case examples illustrate how CR nested within larger, holistic programs of psychiatric rehabilitation can help increase the likelihood of consequential changes in key areas of life function that are of central importance to consumers, family members, and health care providers. These novel approaches to combination treatments that include CR have the potential to permit clinical service providers to enhance their offerings by improving both key objective measures of life function and subjective indices of self-efficacy and life satisfaction in groups of clients historically recalcitrant to both treatment participation and benefit.

## REFERENCES

Barlati, S., Deste, G., De Peri, L., Ariu, C., & Vita, A. (2013). Cognitive remediation in schizophrenia: Current status and future perspectives. *Schizophrenia Research and Treatment*, 2013, 156084.

Bell, M. D., & Bryson, G. (2001). Work rehabilitation in schizophrenia: Does cognitive impairment limit improvement? *Schizophrenia Bulletin*, 27(2), 269–279.

Bell, M. D., Bryson, G., Greig, T., Corcoran, C., & Wexler, B. E. (2001). Neurocognitive enhancement therapy with work therapy. *Archives of General Psychiatry*, 58, 763–768.

Bell, M. D., Bryson, G. J., Greig, T., Fiszdon, J. M., & Wexler, B. E. (2005). Neurocognitive enhancement therapy with work therapy: Vocational outcomes at 6 and 12-months follow-ups. *Journal of Rehabilitation and Research Development*, 42, 829–838.

Bell, M. D., Zito, W., Greig, T., & Wexler, B. E. (2008). Neurocognitive enhancement therapy with vocational services: Work outcomes at two-year follow-up. *Schizophrenia Research*, 195, 18–29.

Bowie, C. R., Gupta, M., Holshausen, K., Jokic, R., Best, M., & Milev, R. (2013). Cognitive remediation for treatment-resistant depression: Effects on cognition and functioning and the role of online homework. *Journal of Nervous and Mental Disease*, 201, 680–685.

Bowie, C. R., McGurk, S. R., Mausbach, B., Patterson, T. L., & Harvey, P. D. (2012). Combined cognitive remediation and functional skills training for schizophrenia: Effects on cognition, functional competence, and real-world behavior. *The American Journal of Psychiatry*, 169, 710–718.

Bracy, O. (1995). *PSS CogRehab, version 95*. Psychological Software Services, Inc., Indianapolis, IN.

Brekke, J. S., Hoe, M., Long, J., & Green, M. F. (2007). How neurocognition and social cognition influence functional change during community-based psychosocial rehabilitation for individuals with schizophrenia. *Schizophrenia Bulletin*, 33, 1247–1256.

Choi, J., & Medalia, A. (2005). Factors associated with a positive response to cognitive remediation in a community psychiatric sample. *Psychiatric Services*, 56, 602–604.

Choi, J., & Medalia, A. (2010). Intrinsic motivation and learning in a schizophrenia-spectrum sample. *Schizophrenia Research*, 118, 12–19.

Cohen, J. (1977). *Statistical power analysis for the behavioral sciences*. New York: Academic Press.

Dickerson, F., Origoni, A., Stallings, C., Khushalani, S., Dickinson, D., & Medoff, D. (2010). Occupational status and social adjustment six months after hospitalization early in the course of bipolar disorder: A prospective study. *Bipolar Disorders*, 12, 10–20.

DiMauro, J., Genova, M., Tolin, D. F., & Kurtz, M. M. (2014). Cognitive remediation for neuropsychological impairment in hoarding disorder. *Journal of Obsessive Compulsive and Related Disorders*, 3, 132–138.

Eack, S. M., Hogarty, G. E., Cooley, S. J., DiBarry, A. L., Hogarty, S. S., Greenwald, D. P., . . . & Keshavan, M. S. (2009). Cognitive enhancement therapy for early-course schizophrenia: Effects of a two-year randomized controlled trial. *Psychiatric Services, 60*(11), 1468–1476.

Eack, S. M., Hogarty, G. E., Greenwald, D. P., Hogarty, S., & Keshavan, M. (2011). Effects of cognitive enhancement therapy on employment outcomes in early schizophrenia: Results from a two-year randomized trial. *Research in Social Work Practice, 21*, 32–42.

Fisher, M., Holland, C., Merzenich, M. M., & Vinogradov, S. (2009). Using neuroplasticity-based auditory training to improve verbal memory in schizophrenia. *American Journal of Psychiatry, 166*, 805–811.

Fisher, M., Holland, C., Subramaniam, K., & Vinogradov, S. (2010). Neuroplasticity-based cognitive training in schizophrenia: An interim report on effects 6-month later. *Schizophrenia Bulletin, 36*, 869–879.

Fiszdon, J. M., Cardenas, A. S., Bryson, G. J., & Bell, M. D. (2005). Predictors of remediation success on a trained memory task. *Journal of Nervous Mental Disease, 193*(9), 602–608.

Fiszdon, J. M., Choi, J., Bryson, G., & Bell, M. D. (2006). Impact of intellectual status on response to cognitive task training in patients with schizophrenia. *Schizophrenia Research, 87*, 261–269.

Green, M. F., Kern, R. S., Braff, D., & Mintz, J. (2000). Neurocognitive deficits and functional outcome in schizophrenia: Are we measuring the "right stuff"? *Schizophrenia Bulletin, 26*(1), 119–36.

Green, M. F., Kern R. S., & Heaton, R. K. (2004). Longitudinal studies of cognition and functional outcome in schizophrenia: Implications for MATRICS. *Schizophrenia Research, 72*(1), 41–51.

Grynszpan, O., Perbal, S., Pelissolo, A., Fossati, P., Jouvent, R., Dubal, S., & Perez-Diaz, F. (2011). Efficacy and specificity of computer-assisted cognitive remediation in schizophrenia: A meta-analytic study. *Psychological Medicine, 41*, 163–173.

Hogarty, G. E., Flesher, S., Ulrich, R., Carter, M., Greenwald, D., Pogue-Geile, M., . . . & Zoretich, R. (2004). Cognitive enhancement therapy for schizophrenia. Effects of a 2-year randomized trial on cognition and behaviour. *Archives of General Psychiatry, 61*, 866–876.

Horan, W. P., Kern, R. S., Tripp, C., Helleman, G., Wynn, J. K., Bell, M., . . . & Green, M. E. (2011). Efficacy and specificity of social cognitive skills training for outpatients with psychotic disorders. *Journal of Psychiatric Research, 45*, 1113–22.

Kern, R. S., Green, M. F., & Satz, P. (1992). Neuropsychological predictors of skills training for chronic psychiatric patients. *Psychiatry Research, 43*, 223–230.

Kontis, D., Huddy, V., Reeder, C., Landau, S., & Wykes, T. (2013). Effects of age and cognitive reserve on cognitive remediation therapy outcome in patients with schizophrenia. *American Journal of Geriatric Psychiatry, 21*, 218–230.

Krabbendam, L., & Aleman, A. (2003). Cognitive rehabilitation in schizophrenia: A quantitative analysis of controlled studies. *Psychopharmacology, 169*, 376–382.

Kurtz, M. M. (2015). Cognitive and social cognitive interventions for schizophrenia. In P. Nathan & J. Gorman (Eds.), *A guide to treatments that work* (4th ed.). New York: Oxford University Press.

Kurtz, M. M., Donato, J., & Rose, J. (2011). Crystallized verbal skills: Relationship to neurocognition, symptoms and functioning in schizophrenia. *Neuropsychology, 25,* 784–791.

Kurtz, M. M., & Gerraty, R. (2009). A meta-analytic investigation of neurocognitive deficits in bipolar illness: Profile and effects of clinical state. *Neuropsychology, 23,* 551–562, 2009.

Kurtz, M. M., Moberg, P. J., Gur, R. C., & Gur, R. E. (2001). Approaches to cognitive rehabilitation in schizophrenia: A review and meta-analysis. *Neuropsychology Review, 11*(4), 197–210.

Kurtz, M. M., & Richardson, C. L. (2012). Social cognitive training for schizophrenia: A meta-analytic investigation of controlled research. *Schizophrenia Bulletin, 38,* 1092–1104.

Kurtz, M. M., Seltzer, J. C., Fujimoto, M., Shagan, D. S., & Wexler, B. E. (2009). Predictors of change in life skills in schizophrenia after cognitive remediation. *Schizophrenia Research, 109,* 267–274.

Kurtz, M. M., Wexler, B. E., Fujimoto, M., Shagan, D. S., & Seltzer, J. C. (2008). Symptoms versus neurocognition as predictors of change in life skills in schizophrenia after outpatient rehabilitation. *Schizophrenia Research, 102,* 303–311, 2008.

Lindenmayer, J. P., McGurk, S. R., Mueser, K. T., Kahn, A., Wance, D., Hoffman, L., . . . & Xie, H. (2008). A randomized controlled trial of cognitive remediation among inpatients with persistent mental illness. *Psychiatric Services, 59,* 241–247.

Lysaker, P. H., Bell, M. D., Zito, W. S., & Bioty, S. M. (1995). Social skills at work: Deficits and predictors of improvement in schizophrenia. *The Journal of Nervous and Mental Disease, 183*(11), 688–692.

McGurk, S. R., & Mueser, K. T. (2006). Cognitive and clinical predictors of work outcomes in clients with schizophrenia receiving supported employment services: 4-Year follow-up. *Administration and Policy in Mental Health and Mental Health Services Research, 33,* 598–606.

McGurk, S. R., Mueser, K. T., Harvey, P. D., LaPuglia, R., & Marder, J. (2003). Cognitive and symptom predictors of work outcomes for clients with schizophrenia in supported employment. *Psychiatric Services, 54*(8), 1129–1135.

McGurk, S. R., Mueser, K. T., & Pascaris, A., (2005). Cognitive training and supported employment for persons with severe mental illness: One-year results from a randomized controlled trial. *Schizophrenia Bulletin, 31,* 898–909.

McGurk, S. R., Twamley, E. W., Sitzer, D. I., McHugo, G. J., & Mueser, K. T. (2007). A meta-analysis of cognitive remediation in schizophrenia. *American Journal of Psychiatry, 164,* 1791–1802.

McKee, M., Hull, J. W., & Smith, T. E. (1997). Cognitive and symptom correlates in participation of social skills training groups. *Schizophrenia Research, 23*(3), 223–229.

Medalia, A., Revheim, N., & Herlands, T. (2009). *Cognitive remediation for psychological disorders: Therapist guide.* New York: Oxford University Press.

Medalia, A., & Richardson, R. (2005). What predicts a good response to cognitive remediation interventions? *Schizophrenia Bulletin 31,* 942–953.

Mueser, K. T., Bellack, A. S., Douglas, M. S., & Wade, J. H. (1991). Prediction of social skill acquisition in schizophrenic and major affective disorder patients from memory and symptomatology. *Psychiatry Research, 37,* 281–296.

Palmer, B. W., Heaton, R. K., Paulsen, J. S., Kuck, J., Braff, D., Harris, M. J., . . . & Jeste, D. V. (1997). Is it possible to be schizophrenic yet neuropsychologically normal? *Neuropsychology, 11*, 437–446.

Penn, D. L., Roberts, D. L., Combs, D., & Sterne, A. (2007). Best practices: The development of the Social Cognition and Interaction Training program for schizophrenia spectrum disorders. *Psychiatric Services, 58*, 449–451.

Pilling, S., Bebbington, P., Kuipers, E., Garety, P., Geddes, J., Orbach, G., . . . & Morgan, C. (2002). Psychological treatments in schizophrenia: II. Meta-analyses of randomized controlled trials of social skills training and cognitive remediation. *Psychological Medicine 32*, 783–791.

Porter R. J., Gallagher, P., Thompson, J. M., & Young, A. H. (2003). Neurocognitive impairment in drug-free patients with major depressive disorder. *British Journal of Psychiatry, 182*, 214–220.

Roberts, D. L., Combs, D. R., Willoughby, M., Mintz, J., Gibson, C., Rupp, B., & Penn, D. L. (2014). A randomized, controlled trial of Social Cognition and Interaction Training (SCIT) for outpatients with schizophrenia spectrum disorders. *British Journal of Clinical Psychology, 53*, 281–298.

Rosen, C., Grossman, L. S., Harrow, M., Bonner-Jackson, A., & Faull, R. (2011). Diagnostic and prognostic significance of Schneiderian first-rank symptoms: A 20-year longitudinal study of schizophrenia and bipolar disorder. *Comprehensive Psychiatry, 52*, 126–131.

Spaulding, W. D., Reed, D., Sullivan, M., Richardson, C., & Weiler, M. (1999). Effects of cognitive treatment in psychiatric rehabilitation. *Schizophrenia Bulletin, 25*, 657–676.

Stevenson, C. S., Whitmont, S., Bornholt, L., Livesey, D., & Stevenson, R. J. (2002). A cognitive remediation programme for adults with Attention Deficit Hyperactivity Disorder. *The Australian and New Zealand Journal of Psychiatry, 36*, 610–616.

Tolin, D. F., Villavicencio, A., Umbach, A., & Kurtz, M. M. (2011). Neuropsychological functioning in hoarding disorder. *Psychiatry Research, 189*, 413–418, 2011.

Twamley, E. W., Jeste, D. V., & Bellack, A. S. (2003). A review of cognitive training in schizophrenia. *Schizophrenia Bulletin, 29*, 359–382.

Twamley, E. W., Vella, L., Burton, C. Z., Heaton, R. K. & Jeste, D. V. (2012). Compensatory cognitive training for psychosis: Effects in a randomized controlled trial. *Journal of Clinical Psychiatry, 73*, 1212–1219.

Van Hulst, B. M., de Zeeuw, P., & Durston, S. (2014). Distinct neuropsychological profiles within ADHD: A latent class analysis of cognitive control, reward sensitivity and timing. *Psychological Medicine, 7*, 1–11.

Wilk, C. M., Gold, J. M., McMahon, R. P., Humber, K., Iaonnone, V. N., & Buchanan, R. W. (2005). No, it is not possible to be schizophrenic yet neuropsychologically normal. *Neuropsychology, 19*, 778–786.

Wykes, T., Huddy, V., Cellard, C., McGurk, S. R., & Czobor, P. (2011). A meta-analysis of cognitive remediation for schizophrenia. *American Journal of Psychiatry, 23*(1), 41–46.

Wykes, T., Reeder, C., Landau, S., Mathiasson, P., Haworth, E., & Hutchinson, C. (2009). Does age matter? Effects of cognitive rehabilitation across the life span. *Schizophrenia Research, 113*, 252–258.

# 2

# Assessment As It Relates to Functional Goals

**PHILIP D. HARVEY AND RICHARD S. E. KEEFE** ■

## INTRODUCTION

The goal of cognitive remediation (CR) therapies is to improve everyday functioning. This goal is met through improving cognition, which then is expected to have an impact on everyday functioning because of the well-understood correlations between cognitive impairments and disability. However, this link is likely not direct, and there are clearly intermediate factors between improved cognition and improved everyday functioning. These factors include the ability to perform the skills required for success in real-world situations, the motivation to perform these skills, and other possible factors interfering with the performance of these skills, such as symptoms and environmental variables. Therefore, assessments of the "true" efficacy of CR approaches need to consider, first, their impact on cognitive performance and second, their impact on functional skills. An additional goal, to ensure that motivation and opportunities are in place to lead to functional success after cognitive enhancement, is addressed in later chapters.

It is important to consider the differences between efficacy (the extent to which a treatment improves a dependent variable in the short term) and effectiveness (the role of a treatment in the outcome of an illness). CR has shown efficacy in short-term clinical trials, but demonstration of effectiveness in the overall treatment of schizophrenia is a critical prerequisite for its widespread adoption as a clinical treatment. Effectiveness information accrues from experience and from research studies to form a combined pool of information about the usefulness of treatments.

In schizophrenia research, use of a standardized battery of neurocognitive, social cognitive, and functional outcomes assessments reduces variability in randomized controlled trials and enhances interpretation of treatment outcome results across research sites (Keefe et al., 2011b). Because it is important that research inform clinical practice, we can draw on empirical data to guide the choice of cognitive assessments for use in a clinical setting. There are, however, a variety of options with respect to measurement of cognitive functioning, including a range of standardized batteries that measure cognitive performance, abbreviated assessments, and interview-based measures of cognitive functioning. Further, CR may be delivered to people with psychological conditions in which cognitive and functional deficits are not as ubiquitous as in schizophrenia. In order to demonstrate the clinical effectiveness of cognitive interventions, it is important to measure improvement in functioning beyond cognition, and this necessitates the selection of additional measures of functional skills and community functioning. This chapter considers how these measures can be used in clinical practice to select patients for CR interventions and to assess their progress during and after cognitive enhancement treatments.

In a clinical setting, the choice of which assessment is most informative may be influenced by a multitude of factors, including resource availability, client characteristics, and the purpose of the assessment. Purposes may include determining individuals' rehabilitation needs, customizing cognitive interventions, and tailoring outcome measures to treatment strategies. Outcome measures can often be crafted or modified based on the treatment targets and the interests of the individual clinician or participant in a treatment intervention or research study. This chapter aims to inform the clinician about the available cognitive and functional assessment options, ranging across both clinical domains and assessment modalities, and to discuss methodological considerations in order to guide the selection of assessments for use in people with schizophrenia in a CR intervention or clinical trial.

## ASSESSMENT OPTIONS IN A CLINICAL SETTING

### Cognitive Performance Batteries

Some clinical service delivery systems routinely provide rehabilitative interventions including CR to target cognition in various neuropsychiatric conditions, and there is increasing interest in the use of pharmacological agents to enhance cognitive functioning (Harvey, 2009; Keefe et al., 2013a). Although the use of validated assessment batteries is standard procedure to determine the efficacy of behavioral or pharmacological interventions in research trials, cognitive assessment can also be valuable in clinical practice. Clinicians and investigators are faced with a variety of assessment strategies from which to choose, as well as potential constraints that can affect the feasibility of implementation. Modalities of cognitive assessment include standardized cognitive batteries, interviews and questionnaires, and co-primary measures of skills related to community functioning. In schizophrenia research, the MATRICS Consensus Cognitive Battery (MCCB) (Nuechterlein et al., 2008), part of the National Institute of Mental Health's Measurement and Treatment Research to Improve Cognition in Schizophrenia (MATRICS) initiative, is the gold standard for cognitive assessment batteries designed to reliably and consistently measure cognitive outcomes in pharmacological treatment trials (Buchanan et al., 2005, 2011). Regulatory authorities also have accepted the MCCB as a final end point for behaviorally based CR interventions.

The MCCB assesses seven domains of cognitive function using ten cognitive tests. These tests were developed largely for neuropsychological or intellectual assessments in general and therefore are sensitive to changes at both low and high ends of the cognitive performance spectrum. Overall, the MCCB has been found to be easy to administer with high fidelity, resulting in very few missing data points even in large, multisite clinical trials (Keefe et al., 2011a). Box 2.1 lists the tests used in the MCCB.

Although the MCCB is certainly the gold standard of measurement, it may be more suitable for use in clinical research trials, which require and accommodate comprehensive assessment batteries to capture a range of potential intervention effects, than for widespread use in clinical settings. The MCCB provides a detailed assessment of a patient's cognitive performance, but in community settings

---

Box 2.1

MATRICS* CONSENSUS COGNITIVE BATTERY: DOMAINS OF FUNCTIONING AND TESTS USED TO CAPTURE THEM

**Speed of Processing**
Category Fluency
Brief Assessment of Cognition in Schizophrenia (BACS)—Symbol-Coding
Trail Making A

**Attention/Vigilance**
Continuous Performance Test—Identical Pairs (CPT-IP)

**Working Memory**
*Verbal*: University of Maryland—Letter-Number Span
*Nonverbal*: Wechsler Memory Scale (WMS)—III Spatial Span

**Verbal Learning**
Hopkins Verbal Learning Test (HVLT)—Revised

**Visual Learning**
Brief Visuospatial Memory Test (BVMT)—Revised

**Reasoning and Problem Solving**
Neuropsychological Assessment Battery (NAB)—Mazes

**Social Cognition**
Meyer-Solovay-Caruso Emotional Intelligence Test

---

*Measurement and Treatment Research to Improve Cognition in Schizophrenia.

resources may be limited. In non-research community clinics, time, space, and financial constraints may preclude staff training on and routine use of comprehensive assessment batteries such as the MCCB for the purposes of treatment planning and outcomes evaluation. Because the MCCB requires approximately 75 minutes of testing time, shorter assessments with similar reliability and validity may be more practical for clinical use. Data from the baseline assessment in the Clinical Antipsychotic Trials of Intervention Effectiveness (CATIE) schizophrenia trial (Keefe, Poe, Walker, Kang & Harvey, 2006c) and targeted studies aimed at the development of abbreviated assessments (Keefe et al., 2004) suggest that a small number of tests or a similarly abbreviated assessment may be sufficient to account for almost all of the variance in the overall cognitive composite score. As shown in Table 2.1, in the CATIE schizophrenia trial, approximately 90% of the variance in a composite score could be accounted for by five tests requiring about 25 minutes of assessment time. Other studies with other samples have generated similar results (Hurford, Marder, Keefe, Reise, & Bilder, 2011; Velligan et al., 2004). An abbreviated assessment has the potential to be a more practical method of assessing treatment change in patients with psychiatric conditions who have been treated with CR, with essentially no reduction in validity of the assessment. Although some assessments are very abbreviated and assess only one or two domains, the results from the CATIE trial suggests that tests measuring processing speed, working and

*Table 2.1.* CORRELATION BETWEEN COMPOSITE PERFORMANCE AND INDIVIDUAL TESTS: CATIE BASELINE SAMPLE ($N = 1035$)

| Variable Entered | Total $R^2$ | $R^2$ Change | Administration Time (min) |
|---|---|---|---|
| WAIS-R Digit Symbol | .610 | .610 | 3.4 |
| HVLT Verbal Memory | .722 | .112 | 4.1 |
| Grooved Pegboard | .790 | .068 | 5.0 |
| Letter-Number Sequencing | .867 | .078 | 5.9 |
| Verbal Fluency | .888 | .021 | 8.0 |
| WISC-R Mazes | .934 | .046 | 11.2 |
| Continuous Performance Test | .956 | .022 | 13.4 |
| Visuospatial Working Memory | .978 | .022 | 16.2 |
| WCST | 1.000 | .022 | 20.0 |

From Keefe, R. S., Bilder, R. M., Harvey, P. D., Davis, S. M., Palmer, B. W., Gold, J. M., . . . & Lieberman, J. A. (2006a). Baseline neurocognitive deficits in the CATIE schizophrenia trial. *Neuropsychopharmacology, 31,* 2003–2046. CATIE = Clinical Antipsychotic Trials of Intervention Effectiveness schizophrenia trial; HVLT = Hopkins Verbal Learning Test; $R^2$ = coefficient of determination; WCST = Wisconsin Card Sorting Test; WISC-R = Wechsler Intelligence Scale for Children–Revised.

episodic memory, and executive functioning can be completed in a very efficient manner. Further, all individual tests have extensive norms that can be used to make decisions regarding the presence of deficits and their improvement with treatment.

The Brief Assessment of Cognition in Schizophrenia (BACS) (Keefe et al., 2004) also offers a feasible assessment alternative that does not involve post hoc selection of tests from a larger battery. Like the MCCB, the BACS measures cognitive functioning in multiple domains of cognition pertinent to schizophrenia. It can be useful in creating a baseline cognitive profile for delineating cognitive treatment targets and informing intervention choices, and it has proven sensitivity for evaluating treatment progress and outcome (Bowie, Grossman, Gupta, Oyewumi, & Harvey, 2014; Bowie, McGurk, Mausbach, Patterson, & Harvey, 2012). The BACS can be administered in 35 minutes and was designed specifically to measure treatment-related changes in cognition in the domains of executive functioning, verbal fluency, verbal memory, working memory, and processing speed. The BACS has alternate forms, thus minimizing practice effects; this is an important consideration for continuous assessment and clinical decision making. Box 2.2 presents the tests contained in the BACS. The BACS has been translated into multiple languages and has been modified for use in patients with mood disorders (Keefe et al., 2014).

Other paper-and-pencil and computerized outcome measures are readily available, such as the Repeatable Battery for the Assessment of Neuropsychological Status (RBANS), CogState, Cambridge Neuropsychological Test Automated Battery (CANTAB), and CNS Vital Signs. Whereas computerized test batteries have the benefit of standardized instructions and the potential to reduce human error, the valid completion rate of computerized test batteries tends to be significantly less than that of pencil-and-paper batteries (Harvey et al., 2013b; Keefe et al., 2006a; Silver et al., 2006). Some computerized methods have not been fully validated and therefore should be used with caution. Many current batteries are not adequately user friendly for neuropsychiatric patients in a clinical setting that does not have trained testing technicians, so they are no more useful than comprehensive neuropsychological assessment batteries.

## Interview-Based Assessment of Cognition

Although cognitive performance measures are the classic measures for assessing cognitive change, several other methods may be acceptable in clinical settings. One method for assessing cognitive change in the clinic uses interview-based measures of cognition that are administered to several different potential informants. A number of interview-based rating scales have become available over the last decade. The Schizophrenia Cognition Rating Scale (SCoRS) (Keefe et al., 2006c) has twenty anchored items rated 1 through 4 that assess all seven MCCB cognitive domains and can be completed in 12 minutes. It is administered separately to patients and to an informant, with cognitive functioning rated in relation to various tasks. Thus, if a patient refuses a cognitive assessment, some information can be obtained from other sources. The interviewer provides a global score based on patient and informant responses and observations of the patient's behavior. Ratings by SCoRS interviewers

Box 2.2

COGNITIVE DOMAINS ASSESSED BY THE BACS*

**Verbal Memory and Learning**
*Verbal Memory:* Patients are presented with fifteen words and then asked to recall as many as possible. This procedure is repeated five times.

**Working Memory**
*Digit Sequencing Task:* Patients are presented with clusters of numbers (e.g., 936) of increasing length. They are asked to tell the experimenter the numbers in order, from lowest to highest.

**Motor Function**
*Token Motor Task:* Patients are given 100 plastic tokens and asked to place them into a container as quickly as possible for 60 seconds using both hands at once.

*Symbol Coding Task:* Patients receive a key explaining how unique symbols correspond to the individual numerals 1 through 9. They are asked to fill in the corresponding number beneath a series of symbols as quickly as possible. There is a 90-second time limit.

**Verbal Fluency**
*Semantic Fluency:* Patients are given 60 seconds to name as many words as possible within a given category.

*Letter Fluency:* In two separate trials, patients are given 60 seconds to generate as many words as possible.

**Executive Function**
*Tower of London:* Patients look at two pictures simultaneously. Each picture shows three colored balls arranged on three pegs, with a unique arrangement of balls in each picture. The patient is asked to give the minimum number of times the balls in one picture would have to be moved to make the arrangement identical to that in the other picture.

*Brief Assessment of Cognition in Schizophrenia.

correlate significantly with performance measures of cognition and account for significant variance in real-world functioning (Keefe et al., 2006c). Similar measures include the Clinical Global Impression of Cognition in Schizophrenia (CGI-CogS) (Ventura, Cienfuegos, Boxer, & Bilder, 2008). In addition, the Cognitive Assessment Interview (CAI) uses items that have the best psychometric characteristics from the CGI-CogS. This ten-item scale can be administered in a very brief period and has been found to have very good statistical and psychometric properties, particularly when clinicians are the informants (Green et al., 2011; Ventura et al., 2013). Figure 2.1 presents sample items from these two scales.

A

# CAI

## Cognitive Assessment Interview

**Joseph Ventura, Robert Bilder, Steve Reise, and Richard Keefe**
**University of California, Los Angeles**
**Semel Institute for Neuroscience and Human Behavior**
**Duke University, Durham, North Carolina**

| DOMAIN: Attention/Vigilance | | |
|---|---|---|
| **3. Problems sustaining concentration over time (without distraction)?** | | |
| *Do you have trouble concentrating? Do you take breaks frequently? Do you have trouble paying attention while reading, listening to the radio or watching television, long enough to read/listen/see a whole article/chapter/program?* | | |
| Patient Examples | Informant Examples | |
| Patient<br>N/A 1  2  3  4  5  6  7 | Informant<br>N/A 1  2  3  4  5  6  7 | Composite<br>N/A 1  2  3  4  5  6  7 |

Contact information: Joseph Ventura, PhD; JVentura@ucla.edu

B

**BASELINE FORM**
**SCHIZOPHRENIA COGNITION RATING SCALE (SCoRS)**

Patient Initials:_____        Patient Randomization Number:_____

Date of Patient Interview:_____  Date of Informant Interview:_____

Informant's Relationship to Patient_____  # of hrs spent with patient per wk_____

Fathers Education Level:_____  Mothers Education Level:_____

The purpose of this questionnaire is to assess problems in attention, memory, motor skills, speech, and problem solving. The questions are designed to measure the patient's severity of cognitive difficulty within the past two weeks. There are a total of 20 questions to be asked of the patient and then the informant in separate interviews. As the interviewer, you will determine your rating based upon your interviews of both the patient and the informant. Please circle the appropriate whole number for each question.

**Level Of Severity**

| N/A = Rating not applicable | 1 = None | 2 = Mild | 3 = Moderate | 4= Severe |
|---|---|---|---|---|

**Do you/Does the patient have difficulty...**

| 1. Remembering names of people you know or meet? | | |
|---|---|---|
| **Example: Roommate, nurse, doctor, family & friends** | | |
| Mild: Remembers most names of people that he/she knows but not all of the people he/she has just met<br>Moderate: Forgets many names of people he/she knows and all of the names of people he/she has just met<br>Severe: Forgets all or almost all names of people he/she knows and meets | | |
| **Patient** | **Informant** | **Interviewer** |
| N/A   1   2   3   4 | N/A   1   2   3   4 | N/A   1   2   3   4 |

Contact information: Richard S.E. Keefe, PhD; Richard.Keefe@duke.edu

**Figure 2.1** A, Sample item from the Cognitive Assessment Interview (CAI). B, Sample item from the Schizophrenia Cognition Rating Scale (SCoRS).

These rating scales enable clinicians to summarize their impressions of the level of cognitive impairment in their patients, either from an interview by a rater or from their own ratings. In randomized studies, these impressions have been shown to be sensitive to the effects of treatment (Harvey, Ogasa, Cucchiaro, Loebel, & Keefe, 2011; Keefe et al., 2015). Such interview-based assessments are practical, are easy to administer, and have high face validity, which makes them useful components of a cognitive and functional assessment. However, they are not a panacea, because patients' self-reports regarding baseline cognitive ability or cognitive change may not have adequate validity (Durand et al., 2015; Keefe et al., 2006b, 2014; see also Chapter 3 in this volume).

For instance, when the SCoRS is administered to patients only, it has low reliability statistics, and the relationship between the SCoRS result and cognitive performance is weak (Keefe et al., 2006c; Keefe et al., 2015). Similar findings have emerged with the CAI: Patient self-reports of their cognitive abilities were found not to correlate with their performance on the MCCB, whereas high-contact clinician ratings were well correlated with cognitive performance, performance on measures of everyday functional skills, and ratings of real-world outcomes (Durand et al., 2015). Further, in the Durand study and others, patient reports were biased by subjective depression, in that patients who self-reported greater severity of depression also reported that they were more cognitively and functionally impaired. Clinician ratings of cognitive deficits did not correlate with patient-reported depression, again raising the question of whether this correlation is a manifestation of response bias. Therefore, the utility of the SCoRS and of CAI depends on the availability of an informant such as a clinician or caregiver to provide information about the patient's cognitive-related behaviors.

The importance of the systematic inclusion of an informant in a comprehensive assessment have been clearly illustrated by the results of several treatment studies. Data from a randomized pharmacological clinical trial investigating the effects of the α-7 nicotinic agonist EVP-6124 suggested that although the interview-based assessment from the SCoRS was sensitive to treatment with EVP-6124 overall, the magnitude of the effect was significantly larger if informants were available to assist in generating the SCoRS ratings (Nutt et al., 2013). When these instruments are used in the clinic, it is important for clinicians to gather information from the correct informants and to consider their own clinical impressions, which in many cases are more accurate than information obtained from other sources, particularly patient self-report.

A important point in the study by Durand et al. (2015) is that clinicians did not receive training in how to generate ratings with the CAI or the real-world functional rating scales used in the study. The rating scales are clearly enough written, easy enough to use, and adequately valid for an experienced clinician to generate ratings that are correlated with objective performance data. Clinicians seeing patients on an everyday basis can trust their impressions of patient functioning if the information is collected on the basis of extended experience with the patients, and this information may be more valuable than that obtained directly from patients' self-reports or from the impressions of their relatives.

There are, however, some limitations to clinician ratings. Clinicians seem most able to generate global impressions of functioning, in both cognitive and functional domains. When asked to make detailed judgments about functioning, such as judging the ability to make assessments of specific functional skills (or specific domains of cognitive deficits), their impressions are less accurate. For instance, in a study in which global clinician ratings of everyday functioning were quite well linked to performance on functional skills tasks, clinicians generated ratings of patients' specific financial skills (e.g., depositing checks, budgeting) that were essentially uncorrelated with direct measures of performance of these skills (Harvey et al., 2013b). Therefore, clinical impression may provide global guidance about functioning but needs to be augmented with direct assessments in many cases.

An additional domain of critical clinical impression is that of the capacity to learn and thus to benefit from CR. Often, referral decisions for CR require consideration of pre-illness levels of cognitive and functional achievement. Individuals with intellectual disability may have reduced potential to benefit from CR interventions, leading to poor progress and substantial frustration on the part of both the client and the treatment staff. This is another area in which direct assessment has considerable potential benefit, because even abbreviated intellectual assessments can detect levels of intellectual disability that might make CR unproductive.

## TREATMENT TARGET CONSIDERATIONS

Many test batteries are sensitive to cognitive deficits in neuropsychiatric conditions and may be considered for use in the assessment of patients receiving CR therapy. The choice of assessment should consider the psychometric properties of the cognitive measures. Overall, composite scores tend to be more sensitive to the cognitive impairments in schizophrenia (Keefe et al., 2011a) and may be used if global cognitive change is the treatment target. Examining relative strengths and weaknesses within a broad cognitive profile provides opportunity to personalize CR training and teach specific strategies to assist in the performance of cognitive skills during activities of daily living.

Clinicians may wish to focus on very specific aspects of cognition to measure the effects of a targeted intervention. For example, it may appear that a patient has a specific deficit in attention, working memory, or problem solving. However, assessment of specific domains of cognition is fraught with psychometric challenges. A focus on a single domain of function truly requires more than a single test. Compared with composite measures, individual tests have lower test-retest reliability, lower correlations with aspects of outcome (McClure et al., 2007), and greater variability; therefore, they have less sensitivity to treatment-related changes (Buchanan et al., 2011; Javitt et al., 2012; Keefe et al., 2011a; Umbricht et al., 2014). Moreover, given that the ultimate goal of CR is generalization, measurement of more than a select set of cognitive domains provides a more comprehensive assessment of clinical effectiveness. A broad-based cognitive assessment offers clinicians the option of examining specific domains as well as overall cognitive gains after treatment. Further, the correlation between cognitive performance and measures of everyday outcomes is substantially greater for composite scores than for any individual domains (Green, Kern, Braff & Mintz, 2000; McClure et al., 2007).

Another challenge of cognitive performance measurements is that some tests are prone to practice effects, and this tendency is variable across tests. Practice-related improvement may be related to familiarity with task content or instructions or procedural learning (Goldberg et al., 2007; Goldberg, Keefe, Goldman, Robinson, & Harvey, 2010). One way of addressing this issue is to use tests with alternate forms, such as verbal learning tests with different word lists. However, tests with alternate forms are particularly vulnerable to reduced test-retest reliability and may not eliminate practice effects completely (Goldberg et al., 2010; Harvey et al., 2005; Keefe et al., 2011a). Variance associated with lack of equivalence between forms is much more difficult to quantify than practice effects because lack of equivalence may affect many different measurement characteristics. Therefore, when a clinician is examining a patient with cognitive performance measures to determine whether treatment has been effective, it is important to take into consideration the expected effects of practice on the measure used. Certain tests with a rule-learning focus, such as the Wisconsin Card Sorting Test (WCST), may be very vulnerable to practice effects and are better measures of baseline impairment than treatment changes. Overall, clinical trial data suggest that the MCCB composite score changes that occur between baseline and follow-up after no treatment or placebo treatment are small, with most studies reporting improvements of less than 0.2 standard deviations (SDs) (Buchanan et al., 2011; Javitt et al., 2012; Keefe et al., 2011a; Umbricht et al., 2014). Therefore, use of a single form of most tests does not lead to any major biases and certainly no ceiling effects in people with schizophrenia.

Making a decision about whether a specific individual has demonstrated change in a cognitive or functional outcome can be difficult. How can a clinician determine whether a certain magnitude of change is caused by treatment or simply by random variation expected in cognitive test performance? One standard method for addressing this issue is the Reliable Change Index, or RCI (Harvey et al., 2005; Heaton et al., 2001; Leifker, Patterson, Bowie, Mausbach, & Harvey, 2010). A standard method for calculating the RCI is to index the expected practice effect plus the 90% confidence interval of the mean change score from baseline to follow-up, which represents the amount of change that will occur only 10% of the time based on random factors unrelated to treatment. For instance, in regard to the MCCB composite score, for which the mean is 50 and the SD is 10, the mean MCCB change with practice is expected to be about 2 T-score points. The SD of this change score is about 6. Therefore, the RCI is $2 + (1.64 \times 6)$, or about 12. This change is slightly greater than 1 SD. If a 12-point change on the MCCB is seen in an individual, the clinician may conclude that 90% of the time this amount of change is definitely nonrandom. This is the same level of change found to be required for reliability in previous batteries that were not fully overlapping with the MCCB (Leifker et al., 2010), suggesting that this may be a reasonable and robust estimate. Although clinical meaning is defined differently by different stakeholders including patients, clinicians, family members, and regulators (Keefe et al., 2013b), this amount of change is likely to be clinically meaningful and is very unlikely to have occurred at random. Clinicians may wish to choose a measure of change that is less conservative—that is, less likely to lead to the erroneous conclusion that a patient is not responding to treatment when in fact he or she is treatment responsive. In the example of the MCCB, this less conservative criterion would define the RCI, indicating clinically meaningful change, as 9 to 10 points.

In one study, CR was compared with a video game control condition in a sample of people with schizophrenia (Keefe et al., 2012). None of the twenty-three patients in the control condition demonstrated a treatment response, but five of the twenty-four patients from the CR condition demonstrated a response of greater than 12 points (1.2 SD) on the MCCB. There are two important implications of these data for our discussion of significant clinical change. First, the number needed to treat in this CR study was five, meaning that one out of five patients treated with CR improved substantially and none of the placebo patients responded. Although this number may seem low, it is actually similar to that widely used for studies of pharmacological treatments for clinical symptoms such as depression. Second, the cognitive gains for subjects whose MCCB scores increased by more than 12 points can be considered clinically meaningful because, as the RCI informs us, an increase of 12 points on the MCCB is unlikely to have occurred by chance, practice, or non–treatment-related variables.

## FUNCTIONAL OUTCOME MEASURES

Although cognitive assessment helps a clinician to understand whether CR is having its expected direct effect on cognitive impairment, improvement in functioning may be a more relevant and desired clinical outcome. One challenge in attempting to demonstrate changes in functional outcomes in patients with severe mental illness is that traditional functional outcome measures, such as job performance, independent living, and social and interpersonal interactions, may be difficult to change over a relatively brief period of time and may be affected by external influences such as disability compensation (Rosenheck et al., 2006). However, performance-based measures of functional *capacity*, such as the UCSD Performance-Based Skills Assessment (UPSA) developed at the University of California, San Diego (Patterson, Goldman, McKibbin, Hughs, & Jeste, 2001a), assess skills related to real-world functioning in the office setting. These performance-based measures show very strong correlations with cognitive outcomes on instruments such as the MCCB, the BACS, and the CogState computerized battery (Green et al., 2011; Harvey et al., 2013a; Keefe et al., 2011a; Keefe, Poe, Walker, & Harvey, 2006b; Pietrzak et al., 2009). Additionally, the UPSA-Brief form is an efficient means of assessing functional capacity that also possesses good psychometric properties (Green et al., 2011; Mausbach, Harvey, Goldman, Jeste, & Patterson, 2007) and has been shown to be sensitive to treatment in CR studies (Bowie et al., 2012). Much as abbreviated cognitive measurements can be suitable for detection of impairment similar to that seen with a long assessment, the abbreviated functional capacity assessments have been shown to be more feasible and as valid as the longer batteries.

There are additional functional capacity measures aimed at social skills (Patterson, Moscona, McKibbin, Davidson, & Jeste, 2001b), medication management (Heaton et al., 2004), and financial skills (Heaton et al., 2004). All of these measures have been found to be related to cognitive performance on the one hand and to real-world functional outcomes on the other, in samples of people with schizophrenia. These functional capacity measures may enable clinicians to determine whether patients are improving in aspects of functional skills that are related to cognition. These instruments are short and address critical aspects of functioning that are required to maintain everyday functioning. Further, they are not dependent on the opportunity to perform skills in the community, which can be an important determinant of real-world outcomes (Holshausen, Bowie, Mausbach, Patterson, & Harvey, 2014). As a result, patients can be assessed for their potential functioning while waiting for the opportunity to make residential or vocational changes. Functional capacity measures also have the benefit of being able to detect improvements in component skills associated with readiness to make functional gains, even in the context of other environmental barriers such as disability compensation.

One of the drawbacks of some of these assessments is that they were designed for patients with functional disability and may not be useful in patients who are functioning relatively well at baseline and have little room to improve on the scale. For such patients, clinicians may choose to measure functional attainment related specifically to the individual's personal goals in social, educational, and vocational domains.

These performance-based assessment measures have been widely used in other conditions, including bipolar disorder, mild cognitive impairment, major depression, post-traumatic stress disorder, and substance abuse. They have been shown to manifest validity in these conditions in that they correlate with both indices of cognitive test performance and measures of real-world everyday functioning. They have also shown practicality in that the measures can be completed in these populations without substantial ceiling effects other than high scores in people with minimal evidence of everyday functional disability.

## Innovations in Functional Capacity Assessment

Historically, functional capacity measures have been composed of paper-and-pencil simulations of everyday tasks or role-playing in manufactured social situations. Recently, several different functional capacity simulations have been developed using computerized strategies. These include virtual reality strategies as well as realistic variants of functional tasks that are already performed on a computer or an equivalent touch-screen device such as an automated teller machine (ATM).

One of these measures, the Virtual Reality Functional Capacity Assessment (VRFCAT; Ruse et al., 2014a, 2014b), has been shown to differentiate schizophrenia patients from healthy controls and to be correlated with paper-and-pencil functional capacity assessments (i.e., UPSA-B) and assessments of cognitive impairment with the MCCB. Figure 2.2 shows screenshots from that task, which involves preparing to cook a meal by developing a shopping list, traveling to and from a grocery store, and shopping. There are several important features of this task other than its relationship to previous measures. These include a structured sequence of tasks and realistic depictions of an apartment, a grocery store, and a transit station. This task is currently administered by an examiner to a single subject, but it is designed to be self-administered so that it could be performed in a waiting room or any other area using a desktop computer.

A second measure is the University of Miami Computerized Assessment Battery (UM CAB). The simulations are in a multimedia format and include graphic representations, video, text, and concurrent speech instructions at a single level of difficulty. They place realistic functional demands on subjects and are objectively scored. Each has multiple alternate forms in English and Spanish. As an added advantage, they can be delivered remotely to subjects. There are several different conditions. *ATM* is a virtual simulation of a banking session. Participants enter

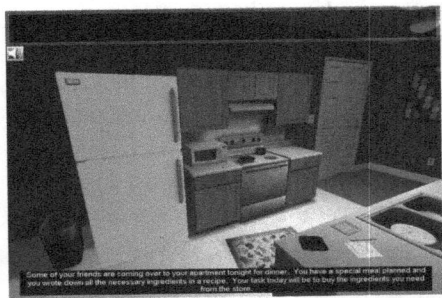
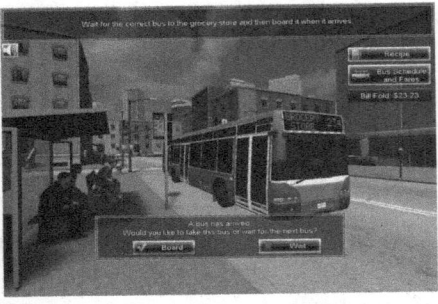
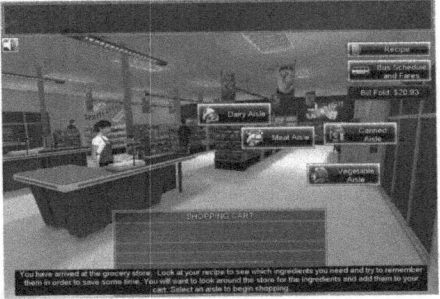

**Figure 2.2** Screenshots from the Virtual Reality Functional Capacity Assessment (VRFCAT).

their personal identification number, check their balance, transfer money, and make a withdrawal. The *Kiosk ticket purchase* is a simulation of a tourist visit to Miami. Participants purchase single-ride and longer-term tickets, check schedules, and add money to their 2-week tourist transit card. *Prescription refill* involves calling a telephone refill service and correctly refilling two prescriptions displayed on the computer screen by entering the prescription numbers, selecting a pickup time, and closing the session. This is a realistic simulation of typical voice menus at commercial pharmacies. *Doctor's visit* is a video interaction with a doctor who writes five prescriptions, provides instructions, and then quizzes the participant about them. The participant also fills a pill organizer with a day's worth of pills, schedules his or her next appointment, and receives instructions on how to prepare for that visit. This assessment battery is based on previous work with healthy older people and has proved capable of separating healthy patients, patients with mild cognitive impairment (MCI), and patients with Alzheimer's disease, as well as differentiating schizophrenia patients from healthy controls. Performance on these simulations is correlated with performance on the MCCB and UPSA-B in both patients and healthy controls. Figure 2.3 shows a screenshot montage from this assessment system.

Computerized functional capacity assessments have shown excellent ability to separate patient groups (e.g., MCI, schizophrenia, bipolar illness) from healthy controls. They have also been shown to produce scores that that are highly related to paper-and-pencil versions of cognitive and functional capacity tests. In the case of simulations of actual computerized tasks (e.g., using an ATM, Internet bill paying), the question of computer familiarity is nicely sidestepped because being able to perform these tests in the everyday world requires the same technology. With other simulations, such as virtual reality doctor's visits and simulated shopping tests, computer or video-game familiarity has the potential to have an effect on performance. These tests have the advantage of being remotely deliverable to individuals who have a computer or tablet, but the requirement for this equipment may limit their use in certain other environments.

## Real-World Functioning

As mentioned at the outset of this chapter, the goal of CR interventions is to improve everyday functioning in a largely disabled population. Although the assessment of everyday functioning may seem straightforward, the problems in self-assessment of cognitive abilities described earlier extend similarly to self-assessment of everyday functioning. Reports by people with schizophrenia tend to manifest very poor convergence with the opinions of other observers and with objective data such as cognitive test or functional capacity performance. Therefore, asking patients about their functioning is not an effective way to obtain valid information about everyday outcomes (Durand et al., 2015). Similar problems have arisen in mood disorders: Individuals with more subjective distress report greater everyday disability in the absence of any objective correlations with performance (e.g., Kaye et al., 2014).

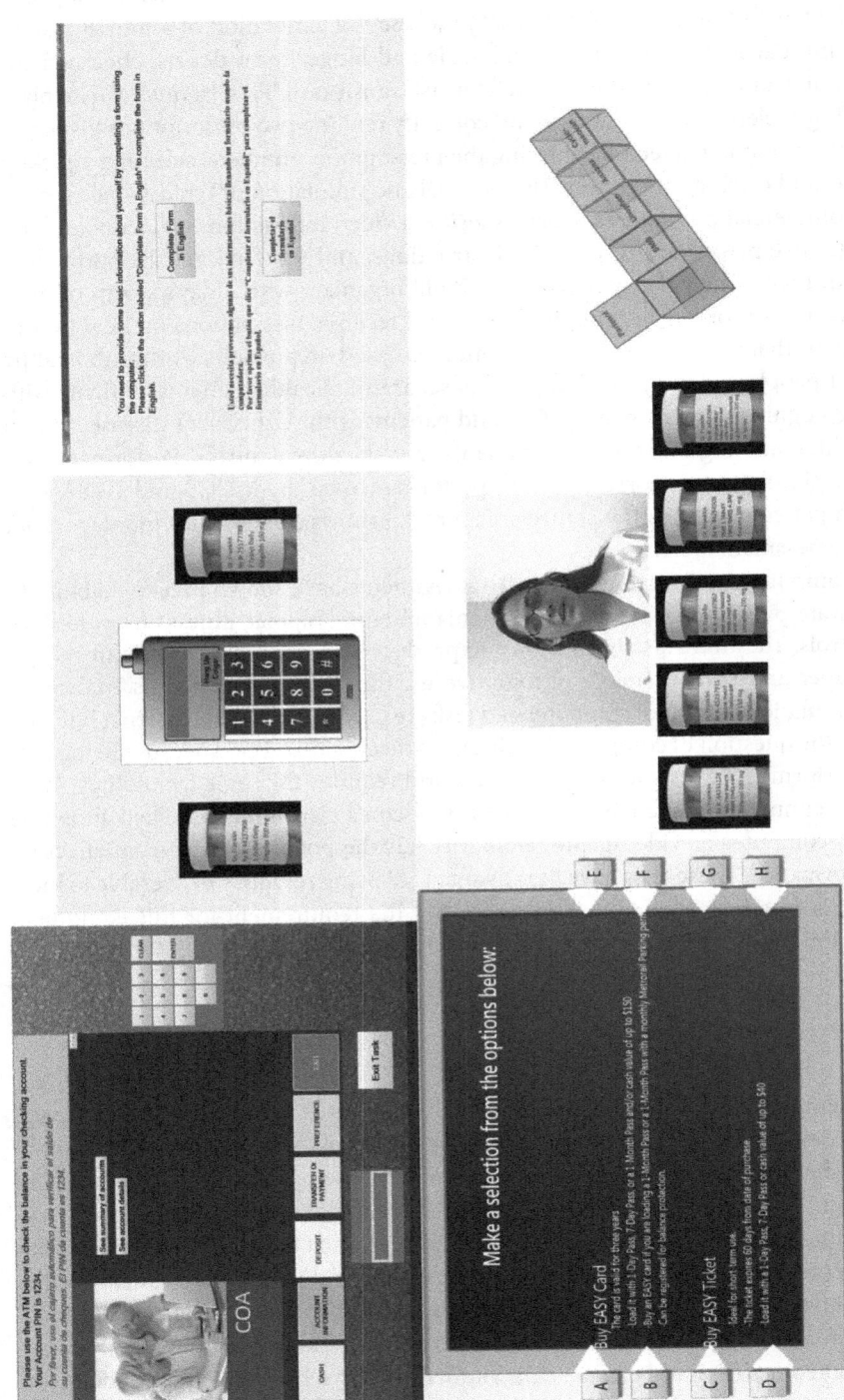

Figure 2.3 Sample tasks from the University of Miami Computerized Assessment Battery.

An alternative strategy involves informant interviews. As discussed earlier, use of informants to generate ratings of cognitive performance leads to increased validity compared with patient self-reports. Choice of informants may be critical, however. In a study that compared patient self-reports, the impressions of high-contact clinicians, and the reports of a friend or relative (Sabbag et al., 2011), there were substantial discrepancies among these sources of information. Self-reports of everyday functioning were not correlated with either friend/relative reports or the impressions of clinicians. Further, reports from friends/relatives and self-reports of everyday functioning were not correlated with scores on tests of functional capacity or cognitive performance. In contrast, although clinicians were unaware of the patients' performance on the tests, clinician impressions were correlated with both cognition and functional capacity scores.

In another analysis of the data from that same sample, patients with schizophrenia who had never been employed in their lives reported that they were more vocationally and socially competent than patients who were currently employed full time (Gould, Sabbag, Durand, Patterson, & Harvey, 2013). At the same time, patients who were working full time or were living independently performed better on objective tests of ability than those who were unemployed or living in supervised settings. These results suggest that objective data regarding ability, which can be collected directly by a clinician through observation, is the best predictor of the likelihood of achievement of functional milestones.

In general, it is difficult to rely on patients' reports of their true levels of potential and achievement. However, in the study by Sabbag et al. (2011), about one third of patients were able to accurately report their functional abilities. There were several predictors of accurate self-assessment as well as predictors of inaccuracy. Patients with higher levels of ability were more likely to be accurate in their self-assessment. An additional predictor of accurate self-assessment was the presence of mild depression. Patients who reported no depression despite their substantially adverse life situations tended to overestimate their cognitive and functional abilities, often substantially. People with higher levels of depression, in the clinical range of moderately severe depression, tended to underestimate their abilities. The presence of psychotic symptoms did not notably affect self-assessment.

## Suggestions for Functional Assessment

As is the case for the assessment of cognitive functioning, the best judge of functioning appears to be the impression of an experienced clinician who knows the patient relatively well and considers all sources of information. Formal ratings may not be required; in our studies, the variance accounted for in accuracy of functional assessments originated from the rater and not the rating scale. Several different rating scales had equivalent validity when rated by a clinician, but none of those scales seemed valid when rated by a friend or relative.

The most critical aspect of functional assessment is an actual focus on functioning as part of ongoing assessments. Our research has shown that clinicians can detect changes in functioning in clinical treatment studies using CR even without training or previous experience with the rating scale. As a result, clinicians may be the single best source of accurate ratings of everyday functioning when they consider all sources of information and know the patient well enough.

## AN ALGORITHM FOR FUNCTIONAL ASSESSMENT

As discussed in this chapter, there are multiple decision points for assessment of the effectiveness of CR on everyday functioning. Performance-based assessments vary in their level of detail and requirements for trained administrators. Ratings require certain types of informants to be adequately valid. Computerized assessments require equipment and space, as well as a trained assessor at times. Coincidently, the research data suggest that the same informants can rate both functioning and cognition and that abbreviated assessments are as valid as longer variants in both cognitive and functional domains. Table 2.2 presents a model that can apply to both cognitive and functional assessments and is viable for use before, during, and after CR interventions.

*Table 2.2.* ASSESSMENT ALGORITHM FOR COGNITIVE
AND FUNCTIONAL ASSESSMENTS

| Test Condition | Cognition | Functioning |
|---|---|---|
| Qualified tester and computers available | Neuropsychological assessment BAC/Short Form NP Assessment Computerized cognitive assessment | Functional capacity testing UPSA/UPSA-B VRFCAT |
| No tester, caregiver available | Interview-based assessment (SCoRS; CAI) | Real-world functioning scales |
| Caregiver unavailable | Interview all possible informants Seek outside clinician input | Interview all possible informants Seek outside clinician input |

BAC = Brief Assessment of Cognition; CAI = Cognitive Assessment Interview; NP = Neuropsychological; SCoRS = Schizophrenia Cognition Rating Scale; UPSA = UCSD Performance-Based Skills Assessment; VRFCA = Virtual Reality Functional Capacity Assessment.

## Interfering Factors

It is also important for clinicians to know what factors may lead to reduced efficacy of CR. Some of these factors are intrinsic to the patient, such as motivation, self-efficacy, and premorbid intellectual and educational attainment; they may be related to other treatments received by the patient if those treatments interfere with the ability to benefit from CR treatments. All of these factors can be measured, and many have been shown to be validly reported by patients, in contrast to patients' ability to self-report and self-assess their functioning.

## Intrinsic Motivation

Motivation to improve in functioning and willingness to engage in activities aimed at self-improvement predict the success of CR interventions. Patients with grossly impaired motivation are probably poor candidates for an effort-oriented intervention such as CR. Intrinsic motivation can be assessed with formal questionnaires but is likely to be easily observed in terms of other aspects of behavior (Choi & Medalia, 2010).

## Self-Efficacy

Patients with high levels of self-efficacy are more likely to manifest real-world functioning consistent with their ability. Self-efficacy is not necessarily a predictor of better real-world functioning; rather, it is an indicator of functioning that is consistent with potential. Patients with low levels of self-efficacy are unlikely to see the connection between exerting effort in a training situation and improving their daily lives (Cardenas et al., 2013; Ho et al., 2013).

## Pharmacological Impediments

It is known that anticholinergic medications interfere with the benefits of CR. Higher daily doses actually negate the benefits of training (Vinogradov et al., 2009). Although similar research has not been performed for antihistamine medication, it has been shown that patients receiving treatment with medications containing high levels of antihistamine binding fail to benefit from practice in cognitive assessments. Both of these classes of medications should probably be carefully monitored.

## Intellectual Functioning

Although most people with neuropsychiatric conditions do not have intellectual functioning in the intellectually disabled range, some do, and the lower IQ on average of people with neuropsychiatric conditions raises the risk that some patients will have low scores. There is no evidence to date that CR raises an individual's IQ, so consideration of the indicators of possible intellectual disability (e.g., low educational attainment, illiteracy) will assist the clinician in not referring patients with very low IQs for a service from which they are unlikely to benefit.

## CONCLUSION

Multiple strategies are available to assess cognitive performance, functional capacity, and real-world outcomes before, during, and after CR therapy. These include short and long cognitive assessments, paper-and-pencil and computerized functional capacity assessments, and interview-based methods. All of these approaches have strengths and weaknesses, but there is considerable evidence of validity and sensitivity across multiple potential outcome measures. The most consistent finding is unreliable self-report on the part of people with neuropsychiatric conditions, which can be obviated with the use of performance-based measures or selection of the correct informant to provide information about a patient's behaviors. There is no reason to believe that different measures should be used for pharmacological cognitive enhancement compared with CR therapy, but this situation could change considerably as more data are obtained from effective pharmacological cognitive enhancement.

The data reviewed in this chapter clearly suggest that for a cognitive and functional assessment to select candidates for CR therapy and to index treatment effects, performance-based assessments are more suitable than self-reported impairments. These assessment strategies have normative data available, allowing for objective identification of patients who need CR and for separation of individuals complaining of cognitive and functional impairment from those who actually meet criteria. These measures allow for detection of change, and both interview- and performance-based measures have been found to be sensitive in CR and pharmacological studies.

## REFERENCES

Bowie, C. R., Grossman, M., Gupta, M., Oyewumi, L. K., & Harvey, P. D. (2014). Cognitive remediation in schizophrenia: Efficacy and effectiveness in patients with early versus long-term course of illness. *Early Intervention in Psychiatry, 8*, 32–38.

Bowie, C. R., McGurk, S. M., Mausbach, B. T., Patterson, T. L., & Harvey, P. D. (2012). Combined cognitive remediation and functional skills training for schizophrenia: Effects on cognition, functional competence, and real-world behavior. *American Journal of Psychiatry, 169*, 710–718.

Buchanan, R. W., Davis, M., Goff, D., Green, M. F., Keefe, R. S. E., Leon, A., ... & Marder, S. (2005). A Summary of the FDA-NIMH-MATRICS workshop on clinical trial designs for neurocognitive drugs for schizophrenia. *Schizophrenia Bulletin, 31*, 5–19.

Buchanan, R. W., Keefe, R. S., Lieberman, J. A., Barch, D. M., Csernansky, J. G., Goff, D. C., . . . & Marder, S.R. (2011). A randomized clinical trial of MK-0777 for the treatment of cognitive impairments in people with schizophrenia. *Biological Psychiatry, 69*, 442–449.

Cardenas, V., Abel, S., Bowie, C. R., Tiznado, D., Depp, C. A., Patterson, T. L., . . . & Mausbach, B. T. (2013). When functional capacity and real-world functioning converge: The role of self-efficacy. *Schizophrenia Bulletin, 39*, 908–916.

Choi, J., & Medalia, A. (2010). Intrinsic motivation and learning in a schizophrenia spectrum sample. *Schizophrenia Research, 118*, 12–19.

Durand, D., Strassnig, M., Sabbag, S., Gould, F., Twamley, E.W., Patterson, T. L., & Harvey, P. D. (2015). Factors influencing self-assessment of cognition and functioning in schizophrenia: Implications for treatment studies. *European Neuropsychopharmacology, 25*, 185–191.

Goldberg, T. E., Goldman, R. S., Burdick, K. E., Malhotra, A. K., Lencz, T., Patel, R. C., . . . & Robinson, D. G. (2007). Cognitive improvement after treatment with second-generation antipsychotic medications in first-episode schizophrenia: Is it a practice effect? *Archives of General Psychiatry, 64*, 1115–1122.

Goldberg, T. E., Keefe, R. S., Goldman, R. S., Robinson, D. G., & Harvey, P. D. (2010). Circumstances under which practice does not make perfect: A review of the practice effect literature in schizophrenia and its relevance to clinical treatment studies. *Neuropsychopharmacology, 35*, 1053–1062.

Gould, F., Sabbag, S., Durand, D., Patterson, T. L., & Harvey, P. D. (2013). Self-assessment of functional ability in schizophrenia: Milestone achievement and its relationship to accuracy of self-evaluation. *Psychiatry Research, 207*, 19–24.

Green, M. F., Kern, R. S., Braff, D. L., & Mintz, J. (2000). Neurocognitive deficits and functional outcome in schizophrenia: Are we measuring the "right stuff"? *Schizophrenia Bulletin, 26*, 119–136.

Green, M. F., Schooler, N. R., Kern, R. S., Frese, F. J., Granberry, W., Harvey, P. D., . . . & Marder, S. R. (2011). Evaluation of functionally meaningful measures for clinical trials of cognition enhancement in schizophrenia. *The American Journal of Psychiatry, 168*, 400–407.

Harvey, P. D. (2009). Pharmacological cognitive enhancement in schizophrenia. *Neuropsychology Review, 19*, 324–335.

Harvey, P. D., Ogasa, M., Cucchiaro, J., Loebel, A., & Keefe, R. S. (2011). Performance and interview-based assessments of cognitive change in a randomized, double-blind comparison of lurasidone vs. ziprasidone. *Schizophrenia Research, 127*, 188–194.

Harvey, P. D., Palmer, B. W., Heaton, R. K., Mohamed, S., Kennedy, J., & Brickman, A. (2005). Stability of cognitive performance in older patients with schizophrenia: An 8-week test-retest study. *The American Journal of Psychiatry, 162*, 110–117.

Harvey, P. D., Siu, C., Hsu, J., Cucchiaro, J., Maruff, P., & Loebel, A. (2013a). Effect of lurasidone on neurocognitive performance in patients with schizophrenia: A short-term placebo- and active-controlled study followed by a 6-month double-blind extension. *European Neuropsychopharmacology, 11*, 1373–1382.

Harvey, P. D., Stone, L., Lowenstein, D., Czaja, S. J., Heaton, R. K., Twamley, E. W., & Patterson, T. L., (2013b). The convergence between self-reports and observer ratings of financial skills and direct assessment of financial capabilities in patients with schizophrenia: More detail is not always better. *Schizophrenia Research, 147*, 86–90.

Heaton, R. K., Marcotte, T. D., Mindt, M. R., Sadek, J., Moore, D. J., Bentley, H., & Grant, I. (2004). The impact of HIV-associated neuropsychological impairment on everyday functioning. *Journal of the International Neuropsychological Society, 10*, 317–331.

Heaton, R. K., Temkin, N., Dikmen, S., Avitable, N., Taylor, M. J., Marcotte, T. D., & Grant, I. (2001). Detecting change: A comparison of three neuropsychological methods, using normal and clinical samples. *Archives of Clinical Neuropsychology, 16*, 75–91.

Ho, J. S., Moore, R. C., Davine, T., Cardenas, V., Bowie, C. R., Patterson, T. L., & Mausbach, B. T. (2013). Direct and mediated effects of cognitive function with multidimensional outcome measures in schizophrenia: The role of functional capacity. *Journal of Clinical and Experimental Neuropsychology, 35*, 882–895.

Holshausen, K., Bowie, C. R., Mausbach, B. T., Patterson, T. L., & Harvey, P. D. (2014). Neurocognition, functional capacity, and functional outcomes: The cost of inexperience. *Schizophrenia Research, 152*, 430–444.

Hurford, I. M., Marder, S. R., Keefe, R. S. E., Reise, S. P., & Bilder, R. M. (2011). A brief cognitive assessment tool for schizophrenia: Construction of a tool for clinicians. *Schizophrenia Bulletin, 37*, 538–545.

Javitt, D. C., Buchanan, R. W., Keefe, R. S. E., Kern, R., McMahon, R. P., Green, M. F., ... & Marder, S. R. (2012). Effect of the neuroprotective peptide davunetide (AL-108) on cognition and functional capacity in schizophrenia. *Schizophrenia Research, 136*, 25–31.

Kaye, J. L., Dunlop, B. W., Iosifescu, D. V., Mathew, S. J., Kelley, M. E., & Harvey, P. D. (2014). Cognition, Functional Capacity, and Self-reported Disability in Women with Posttraumatic Stress Disorder: Examining the Convergence of Performance Based Measures and Self Reports. *Journal of Psychiatric Research, 57*, 51–57.

Keefe, R. S., Bilder, R. M., Harvey, P. D., Davis, S. M., Palmer, B. W., Gold, J. M., ... & Lieberman, J. A. (2006a). Baseline neurocognitive deficits in the CATIE schizophrenia trial. *Neuropsychopharmacology, 31*, 2033–2046.

Keefe, R. S., Buchanan, R. W., Marder, S. R., Schooler, N. R., Dugar, A., Zivkov, M., & Stewart, M. (2013a). Clinical trials of potential cognitive-enhancing drugs in schizophrenia: What have we learned so far? *Schizophrenia Bulletin, 39*, 417–435.

Keefe, R. S., Davis, V. G., Spagnola, N. B., Hilt, D., Dgetluck, N., Ruse, S., ... & Harvey, P. D. (2015). Reliability, validity and treatment sensitivity of the Schizophrenia Cognition Rating Scale. *European Neuropsychopharmacology, 25*, 176–184.

Keefe, R. S., Fox, K. H., Davis, V. G., Kennel, C., Walker, T. M., Burdick, K. E., & Harvey, P. D. (2014). The Brief Assessment of Cognition in Affective Disorders (BAC-A): Performance of patients with bipolar depression and healthy controls. *Journal of Affective Disorders, 166*, 86–92.

Keefe, R. S., Fox, K. H., Harvey, P. D., Cucchiaro, J., Siu, C., & Loebel, A. (2011a). Characteristics of the MATRICS consensus cognitive battery in a 29-site antipsychotic schizophrenia clinical trial. *Schizophrenia Research, 125*, 161–168.

Keefe, R. S., Goldberg, T. E., Harvey, P. D., Gold, J. M., Poe, M., & Coughenour, L. (2004). The Brief Assessment of Cognition in Schizophrenia: Reliability, sensitivity, and comparison with a standard neurocognitive battery. *Schizophrenia Research, 68*, 283–297.

Keefe, R. S., Kraemer, H. C., Epstein, R. S., Frank, E., Haynes, G., Laughren, T. P., ... & Leon, A. C. (2013b). Defining a clinically meaningful effect for the design and interpretation of randomized controlled trials. *Innovations in Clinical Neuroscience, 10,* 4S–19S.

Keefe, R. S., Poe, M., Walker, T. M., & Harvey, P. D. (2006b). The relationship of the Brief Assessment of Cognition in Schizophrenia (BACS) to functional capacity and real-world functional outcome. *Journal of Clinical and Experimental Neuropsychology, 28,* 260–269.

Keefe, R. S., Poe, M., Walker, T. M., Kang, J. W., & Harvey, P. D. (2006c). The Schizophrenia Cognition Rating Scale (SCoRS): Interview-based assessment and its relationship to cognition, real-world functioning and functional capacity. *The American Journal of Psychiatry, 163,* 426–432.

Keefe, R. S., Vinogradov, S., Medalia, A., Buckley, P. F., Caroff, S. N., D'Souza, D. C., . . . & Stroup, T. S. (2012). Feasibility and pilot efficacy results from the multi-site Cognitive Remediation in the Schizophrenia Trials Network (CRSTN) study. *Journal of Clinical Psychiatry, 73,* 1016–1022.

Keefe, R. S., Vinogradov, S., Medalia, A., Silverstein, S. M., Bell, M. D., Dickinson, D., . . . & Stroup, T. S. (2011b). Report from the working group conference on multi-site trial design for cognitive remediation in schizophrenia. *Schizophrenia Bulletin, 37,* 1057–1065.

Leifker, F. R., Patterson, T. L., Bowie, C. R., Mausbach, B. T., & Harvey, P. D. (2010). Psychometric properties of performance-based measurements of functional capacity. *Schizophrenia Research, 119,* 246–252.

Mausbach, B. T., Harvey, P. D., Goldman, S. R., Jeste, D. V., & Patterson, T. L. (2007). Development of a brief scale of everyday functioning in persons with serious mental illness. *Schizophrenia Bulletin, 33,* 1364–1372

McClure, M. M., Bowie, C. R., Patterson, T. L., Heaton, R. K., Weaver, C., Anderson, H., & Harvey, P. D. (2007). Correlations of functional capacity and neuropsychological performance in older patients with schizophrenia: Evidence for specificity of relationships? *Schizophrenia Research, 89,* 330–338.

Nuechterlein, K. H., Green, M. F., Kern, R. S., Baade, L. E., Barch, D. M., Cohen, J. D., . . . & Marder, S. R. (2008). The MATRICS Consensus Cognitive Battery, part 1: Test selection, reliability, and validity. *The American Journal of Psychiatry, 165,* 203–213.

Nutt, D., Gispen de Wied, C. C., Arango, C., Keefe, R. S. E., Penades, R., . . . & Sahakian, B. J. (2013). Cognition in schizophrenia: Summary Nice Consultation Meeting 2012. *European Neuropsychopharmacology, 23,* 769–778.

Patterson, T. L., Goldman, S., McKibbin, C. L., Hughs, T., & Jeste, D. V. (2001a). UCSD Performance-Based Skills Assessment: Development of a new measure of everyday functioning for severely mentally ill adults. *Schizophrenia Bulletin, 27,* 235–245.

Patterson, T. L., Moscona, S., McKibbin, C. L., Davidson, K., & Jeste, D. V. (2001b). Social skills performance assessment among older patients with schizophrenia. *Schizophrenia Research, 48,* 351–360.

Pietrzak, R. H., Olver, J., Norman, T., Piskulic, D., Maruff, P., & Snyder, P. J. (2009). A comparison of the CogState Schizophrenia Battery and the Measurement and Treatment Research to Improve Cognition in Schizophrenia (MATRICS) Battery in assessing cognitive impairment in chronic schizophrenia. *Journal of Clinical and Experimental Neuropsychology, 31,* 848–859.

Rosenheck, R., Leslie, D., Keefe, R., McEvoy, J., Swartz, M., Perkins, D., . . . & CATIE Study Investigators Group. (2006). Barriers to employment for people with schizophrenia. *The American Journal of Psychiatry, 163,* 411–417.

Ruse, S. A., Davis, V. G., Atkins, A. S., Krishnan, K. R., Fox, K. H., Harvey, P. D., & Keefe, R. S. (2014a). Development of a virtual reality assessment of everyday living skills. *Journal of Visualized Experiments, 86*, 51405.

Ruse, S. A., Harvey, P. D., Davis, V. G., Atkins, A. S., Fox, K. H., & Keefe, R. S. (2014b). Virtual reality functional capacity assessment in schizophrenia: Preliminary data regarding feasibility and correlations with cognitive and functional capacity performance. *Schizophrenia Research: Cognition, 1*, e21-e26.

Sabbag, S., Twamley, E. M., Vella, L., Heaton, R. K., Patterson, T. L., & Harvey, P. D. (2011). Assessing everyday functioning in schizophrenia: Not all informants seem equally informative. *Schizophrenia Research, 131*, 250–255.

Silver, J. M., Koumaras, B., Chen, M., Mirski, D., Potkin, S. G., Reyes, P., . . . & Gunay, I. (2006). The effects of rivastigmine on cognitive function in patients with traumatic brain injury. *Neurology, 67*, 748–755.

Umbricht, D., Keefe, R., Murray, S., Lowe, D., Porter, R., Garibaldi, G., & Santarelli, L. (2014). A randomized, placebo-controlled study investigating the nicotinic α7 agonist, RG3487, for cognitive deficits in schizophrenia. *Neuropsychopharmacology, 39*, 1568–1577.

Velligan, D. I., DiCocco, M., Bow-Thomas, C. C., Cadle, C., Glahn, D. C., Miller, A. L., . . . & Crismon, M. L. (2004). A brief cognitive assessment for use with schizophrenia patients in community clinics. *Schizophrenia Research, 71*, 273–283.

Ventura, J., Cienfuegos, A., Boxer, O., & Bilder, R. (2008). Clinical global impression of cognition in schizophrenia (CGI-CogS): Reliability and validity of a co-primary measure of cognition. *Schizophrenia Research, 106*, 59–69.

Ventura, J., Reise, S. P., Keefe, R. S. E., Hurford, I. M., Wood, R. C., & Bilder, R. M. (2013). The Cognitive Assessment Interview (CAI): Reliability and validity of a brief interview-based measure of cognition. *Schizophrenia Bulletin, 39*, 583–591.

Vinogradov, S., Fisher, M., Warm, H., Holland, C., Kirshner, M. A., & Pollock, B. G. (2009). The cognitive cost of anticholinergic burden: Decreased response to cognitive training in schizophrenia. *American Journal of Psychiatry, 166*, 1055–1062.

# 3

# Treatment Planning

## ALICE SAPERSTEIN AND ALICE MEDALIA ■

## INTRODUCTION

The ultimate goals of cognitive remediation are to help individuals attain personal rehabilitation goals and to support their success in the community. Cognitive remediation (CR) does this by improving the cognitive abilities that underlie learning and adaptive functioning in real-world contexts. CR is a behavioral intervention that becomes recovery oriented when it is personalized and integrated into a psychosocial treatment plan that addresses client-initiated recovery goals. In this way, the cognitive goals identified in a CR treatment plan are personally and meaningfully linked to everyday life for each individual. The purpose of this chapter is to guide the clinician through the components and process of treatment planning for CR as a recovery-oriented practice.

## EMPIRICAL BASIS FOR COGNITIVE REMEDIATION TREATMENT PLANNING

The treatment planning strategies discussed in this chapter are based on empirical data supporting restorative-based training and strategy-based approaches to CR. At its core, CR is a skill-learning intervention that capitalizes on the capacity for neuroplasticity and neurogenesis (Kaneko & Keshavan, 2012; Medalia & Choi, 2009). Through regular, repeated, targeted cognitive exercise, neuroanatomical connections may be strengthened and/or repaired, yielding positive changes in neuropsychological abilities. Empirical evidence for this therapeutic mechanism in schizophrenia is suggested by data showing that patients receiving CR demonstrated a decelerated loss, and in some cases an increase, in gray matter volume that was associated with improved cognition (Eack et al., 2010). When the cognitive skill learning occurs in an environment that encourages use of skills and adaptive strategies, clients are helped to further capitalize on brain malleability and ultimately improve their functioning (Bowie, McGurk, Mausbach, Patterson, & Harvey, 2012; Spaulding, Sullivan, & Poland, 2003). This has implications for the context in which CR is carried out (e.g., within a broader psychosocial rehabilitation program).

The CR clinician can devise a program of restorative cognitive training to target skills ranging from visual/auditory information processing, attention, and processing speed to working memory, verbal learning, reasoning, and problem-solving skills. Massed practice consists of repeated cognitive exercise at least two to three times weekly to encourage retention and application of the skills developed. Restorative approaches targeting basic neurocognitive skills are commonly paired with metacognitive exercises to help the individual place cognitive processes within a personally meaningful context, to aid abstraction, and to assist the individual to devise strategies for completing everyday cognitive tasks (Hogarty & Flesher, 1999; Medalia, Revheim, & Herlands, 2009; Wykes & Reeder, 2005). All of these approaches to CR involve skill learning and can be used in either an individual or a group setting.

A fundamental element of recovery-oriented CR for schizophrenia is the tailoring of a treatment plan to suit the specific needs of the individual. This is a fluid, continuous process; as needs change, the treatment plan can be altered. Baseline assessment of cognitive functioning, learning style, and functional goals informs the initial plan, and ongoing tracking of in-session performance and goal attainment facilitates modifications to the treatment plan. Thus, based on an individual's cognitive profile, learning needs, and unique recovery goals, training exercises may be selected to target specific cognitive abilities. Appropriate information processing strategies and skills to facilitate learning and adaptive functioning can be taught. By incorporating CR goals into a broader recovery-oriented rehabilitation plan, cognitive learning may be supported and reinforced by the client's treatment team. Providing CR in an integrative, recovery- and goal-oriented setting has the effect of enhancing the durability and generalizability of therapeutic gains and facilitating an individual's progress toward functional recovery.


## ASSESSMENT

Assessment for CR treatment planning is the first formal opportunity for a CR therapist to form a case conceptualization and to begin cultivating a working alliance. The initial assessment meeting is an appropriate time to orient the client toward the purpose and structure of CR, and it also provides a context for the subsequent assessment procedures. During the initial assessment, the therapist ascertains the client's learning history, evaluates potential barriers to learning, defines areas of relative cognitive strength and weakness through structured cognitive evaluation, assesses perceived cognitive problems, and discusses the client's current recovery goals. The learning history can include the number of years of education, successes in school or in the workplace, and struggles in school or in the workplace. The therapist may ask about any history of learning disability, attention-deficit hyperactivity disorder, or special education. A brief reading test such as the Wechsler Test of Adult Reading (Holdnack, 2001) or the Wide Range Achievement Test—Reading Subtest (Wilkinson & Robertson, 2006), completed as a part of the cognitive evaluation, can provide an estimate of intellectual functioning (i.e., Full Scale IQ) (Griffin, Mindt, Rankin, Ritchie, & Scott, 2002) and indicate the client's reading ability. An IQ estimate is helpful for ruling out intellectual disability and for determining the individual's pre-illness cognitive capacity, against which current cognitive ability can be compared. Assessment of reading also reveals the degree of assistance the client may require to comprehend exercise instructions and materials used throughout the course of CR.

Although most people with mental disorders such as psychotic and mood disorders have problems with attention, memory, and problem solving, the relative degrees of these deficits and the ways in which they manifest differ from person to person. Having a client perform a set of standardized cognitive tests provides two types of information that are helpful for getting to know the client's treatment needs. First, cognitive assessment helps the therapist identify the areas of cognition that require more or less intensive practice. Second, behavioral observations made during the assessment illustrate how the individual approaches cognitive tasks, which likely reflects how tasks and novel situations are approached in other environments as well. The reader may refer to Chapter 2 of this volume to learn more about methods of cognitive assessment that are informative and feasible for routine clinical practice. Use of data derived from the assessment for treatment planning purposes is described here.

Objective tests of cognition yield standardized scores, often expressed as either T-scores or Z-scores, which allow the therapist to compare the client's cognitive performance with that of the normative comparison population. Comparing the standardized score from each cognitive ability test with that of the reading test clarifies the difference between current cognitive functioning and estimated intellectual ability (Figs. 3.1 and 3.2). Taking these data together, the therapist learns

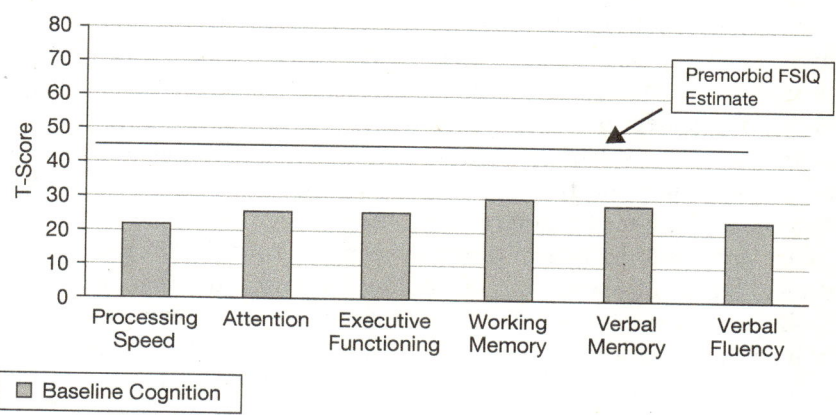

**Figure 3.1** Cognitive performance profile—client A. FSIQ = Full Scale IQ.

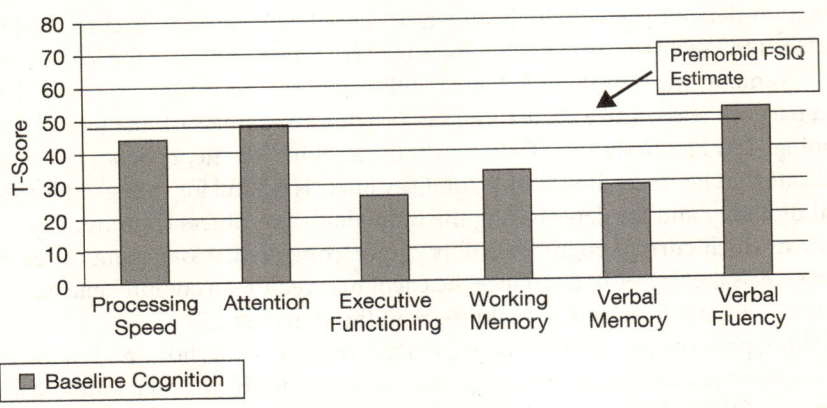

**Figure 3.2** Cognitive performance profile—client B. FSIQ = Full Scale IQ.

how the client is performing on cognitive tests relative to age-matched healthy individuals and to the client's own pre-illness ability. For example, a T-score of 50 (50th percentile, or average) on a test of working memory would not indicate impairment relative to the general population but would indicate impairment if the client's pre-illness ability were in the superior range. The cognitive profile generated from a client's performance on an assessment battery elucidates his or her unique strengths and weaknesses and provides the basis for formulating an initial list of cognitive targets and the exercises that can be used in a restorative training capacity. Behavioral observations made during the assessment may provide the basis for formulating initial learning goals and thereby set the stage for effective cognitive skill learning to take place.

In addition to assessing cognition, the CR therapist should inquire about the client's recovery goals, such as goals regarding socialization, independent living, work, or school. This provides a context for discussing perceived cognitive difficulties and for framing the CR treatment plan. Specifically, areas of cognitive difficulty may be pinpointed as barriers to goal achievement. For example, Client A may report, "I have trouble keeping up with conversation and staying focused when I'm with a group of people. This makes it hard for me to be social with friends and family." With Client A, slow processing speed and impaired attention are evident on objective measures of neurocognition (see Fig. 3.1) and, according to this self-report, impose a barrier to achieving a socialization goal. Client B may report, "I can't remember which pills I've taken when I'm doing my morning medication routine. I need to be able to manage my meds independently in order to get my own apartment." For Client B, poor memory is evident on objective measures of working memory and verbal memory (see Fig. 3.2) and is experienced as a significant obstacle to achieving an independent living goal. These examples illustrate how objective indicators of cognitive deficit combined with self-report of cognitive problems can inform cognitive targets that, with improvement, will yield meaningful changes in real-world functioning.

Sharing these data with the client's treatment team helps other providers understand the cognitive context in which each individual operates and defines the role of CR as an integrated treatment component in the service of the individual's goals for recovery. It behooves the treatment team to know that memory impairment—as opposed to nonadherence, for example—is hindering Client B's ability to independently manage medications. Together, the team can provide adaptive strategies, in combination with memory training, to improve functioning.

Finally, the initial assessment is an opportunity to address clients' questions or concerns about participating in CR. For some, this may include trepidation about using a computer or navigating Web-based cognitive programs. A brief evaluation of facility of computer use (e.g., familiarity with mouse, keyboard, and Internet use) may be warranted. This may yield vital information to help the clinician choose appropriate cognitive exercises and plan the initial session. For some, an introductory lesson on computer use may be needed.

## FORMULATING THE INITIAL PLAN

There are several elements that can be incorporated into an individualized CR treatment plan, including cognitive targets identified from the baseline cognitive profile, recommended cognitive exercises, initial learning goals to help optimize the client's learning potential, references to the client's goals for recovery, and objectives to tie CR to the overall recovery plan. Examples of treatment plans are depicted in Figures 3.3 and 3.4.

Whereas cognitive targets are determined primarily by the cognitive profile, recommended cognitive exercises are carefully selected by the therapist. Choosing

---

**Recovery Plan Goal:** *To improve communication skills and increase socialization*

**Cognitive Remediation Objectives:**
1. *Client A will practice responding quickly to important information needed to complete tasks at hand.*
2. *Client A will identify sources of distraction and develop strategies for staying focused in conversations to improve communication and social skills*

| **Initial Cognitive Targets:**<br>1. *Processing Speed*<br>2. *Selective Attention*<br>3. *Flexible Attention*<br><br>**Recommended Cognitive Exercises:**<br>Program A: *Exercise 1*<br>          *Exercise 2*<br>          *Exercise 3*<br><br>Program B: *Exercise 1*<br>          *Exercise 2*<br>          *Exercise 3* | **Initial Learning Goals:**<br>1. *Practice staying on task for 10 minutes at a time*<br>2. *Increase awareness of when distraction occurs*<br>3. *Identify 3 distracters that impact attention and learning* |
|---|---|

**Figure 3.3** Treatment Plan, Client A

**Recovery Plan Goal**: *To get my own apartment*

**Cognitive Remediation Objectives:**
1. *Client B will practice carrying out mental manipulations using information in memory*
2. *Client B will practice maintaining verbal and visual information in memory in the face of distraction.*
3. *Client B will develop strategies to encode and recall information needed to complete activities of daily living*

| Initial Cognitive Targets: | Initial Learning Goals: |
|---|---|
| 1. *Working Memory*<br>2. *Visual Memory*<br>3. *Verbal Learning*<br><br>**Recommended Cognitive Exercises:**<br>Program A: *Exercise 1*<br>      *Exercise 2*<br>      *Exercise 3*<br>Program B: *Exercise 1*<br>      *Exercise 2*<br>      *Exercise 3* | 1. *Aim to be on-time for CR 50% of sessions*<br>2. *Use session notes to practice setting up learning activities independently*<br>3. *Identify exercises that are most engaging and valuable* |

**Figure 3.4** Treatment Plan, Client B

an appropriate starting place for cognitive exercise is important because the client needs to be provided with an appropriate level of cognitive challenge. As seen in Figure 3.3, Client A, who exhibits slow processing speed and poor attention, will begin training on more focal cognitive exercises for speed, selective attention, and flexible attention; beginning with exercises that focus more on complex cognitive skills such as problem solving might prove too challenging and cause unneeded frustration. In contrast, Client B (see Fig. 3.4) will begin with training tasks that target working memory, visual memory, and verbal learning. Because exercises typically do not isolate one cognitive domain to the exclusion of others, Client B will also likely practice speed and attention while executing the memory tasks. The treatment plans for Clients A and B show how the selected exercises differ in their relative cognitive focus and task complexity. By personalizing the area of cognitive focus, each client also gains practice in the use of strategies to aid information processing and task completion. Together, those cognitive skills and compensatory strategies will be appropriate for each individual's baseline cognitive profile and relevant for his or her recovery goals.

When formulating the initial treatment plan, the CR therapist should consider employing multiple exercises that target a discrete set of cognitive skills. A general guideline is to provide practice on three to four Web-based exercises in each 60-minute session, with 10 to 15 minutes devoted to each exercise. Problem-solving exercises may require more time (15 to 20 minutes), meaning that fewer exercises would be practiced in any given session. Ideally, the choice of exercises within each session should be complementary, so that similar skill sets are practiced in different ways, and consistent with the cognitive targets identified in the initial training plan. When a client is practicing a skill set, task mastery is not necessary for progression from one exercise to the next. Rather, because the exercises are complementary, skills and strategies developed from other exercises may be newly applied to tasks previously practiced, thereby reinforcing what has been learned and promoting a sense of competency for task completion.

In addition, although tasks may target a similar skill set, some task properties may differentially impact a client's engagement and learning. Observing a client practicing a cognitive skill in multiple exercise contexts helps the therapist fine-tune the selection of cognitive exercises in the initial training plan as well as the conceptualization of the client's learning needs. In a group with six to eight clients and one clinician, observation can be accomplished by walking around the room while clients are working at their tasks and watching each group member for several minutes. The goal is to identify the types of learning activities that engage, motivate, and appropriately challenge each client to learn. Table 3.1 lists examples of task properties that may suit different learning needs.

*Table 3.1.* PROPERTIES OF COGNITIVE EXERCISES THAT MAY SUIT DIFFERENT LEARNING NEEDS

| Property | Examples |
|---|---|
| Method of response | Keyboard<br>Mouse control<br>Typing and spelling |
| Adaptability of cognitive challenge | Level of difficulty is uniform throughout the exercise.<br>Level of difficulty is on a continuum. |
| Degree of user control | Task properties are modulated by the program.<br>User can control task parameters to personalize the cognitive exercise. |
| Contextualization | The exercise reflects real-world use of cognitive skills and strategies.<br>Context is artificial. |
| Presentation | Exercise is two-dimensional and sensory limited.<br>Exercise is three-dimensional and multisensory. |
| Goal properties | Goals are proximal, requiring performance of a limited set of operations to complete a task.<br>Goals are distal, requiring multiple steps in sequence to complete a task. |
| Performance feedback | Task offers continuous real-time feedback on performance.<br>Task provides feedback summary on task completion. |
| User assistance | Exercise offers hints to facilitate task progress.<br>Exercise provides strategies for use in subsequent trials.<br>No coaching is provided. |

There is additional therapeutic value in providing multiple exercises to target an area of cognition within the initial stages of treatment planning. Providing clients opportunities for choice among a set of learning activities promotes a sense of autonomy, or self-determination, which can have the effects of enhancing motivation to perform the task itself and facilitating a working alliance between therapist and client (Ryan & Deci, 2000). Fostering intrinsic motivation in the early stages of CR benefits the client by enhancing initial engagement and may set the stage for a longer-term commitment and persistence throughout the learning process.

During the initial assessment and treatment planning stages, it is important for the therapist to view his or her role as not only cognitive coach but also teacher. Because CR is a learning-based intervention, there is an educational focus to the treatment plan. Information gathered from the baseline assessment regarding successes and challenges in other life domains (e.g., work, school) and behavioral observations of task approach and performance may inform the delineation of additional learning goals. In the context of cognitive practice, the client will develop skills and competencies to become an effective learner and to overcome barriers that may impede progress on recovery goals.

In the initial stage of treatment, learning goals may be oriented toward building a context for CR and engaging the client in treatment. Goals may be psychoeducational in nature, helping the client learn about cognition and the role of cognitive skills in everyday life, or they may be insight oriented, helping the client to develop an awareness of cognitive problems and the skills and strategies that can be learned to overcome them. Goals may relate to improving learning behavior, such as regular and/or timely attendance at CR sessions, practice staying on task for incremental lengths of time, or identifying learning preferences and needs to build an effective personalized learning environment. In addition to helping the client develop skills as an effective learner, gradually increased independence in CR may further promote a sense of competency, motivation, and persistence. Like cognitive goals, learning goals will change as progress is made over time.

## THE ROLE OF ONGOING ASSESSMENT

During the initial stages of CR, the clinician maps out a preliminary plan of cognitive targets based on the individual's cognitive profile, cognitive complaints, and recovery goals. The initial treatment plan also includes goals for fostering treatment engagement and building motivation. When used within the CR session, the treatment plan becomes a dynamic document that can be modified based on the therapist's ongoing assessment of an individual's cognitive gains, motivation, and learning needs. Continuous observation of the client's performance guides subsequent training decisions with respect to the choice of cognitive exercises and the pacing of exercise progression. As clients become more confident in their ability to master the initial level of cognitive challenge, the clinician can alter the task parameters to increase task complexity. Once clients become familiar with the software program, they may work with the therapist and begin to exercise more control over the parameters to provide an appropriate level of challenge.

For example, some programs allow users to control time constraints. Whereas turning a timer off may be helpful in the beginning to promote mastery of one cognitive task, adding a timed component, which can sometimes be done gradually or in increments, allows the client to progressively increase the level of challenge by adding another cognitive skill (e.g., processing speed). Alternatively, some software programs employ a learning algorithm that adapts the level of task difficulty based on the client's performance, thereby providing continuously challenging, dynamic cognitive training (Merzenich, Van Vleet, & Nahum, 2014). Task parameters are typically modulated with respect to timing, addition of distracters, and cognitive load. If the training exercise does not automatically adjust to the level of the user's performance, it is important for the therapist to monitor clients' performance, gauging task performance as well as task approach. If a client disengages from the training session, the therapist should work with that client to discern whether the task is still appropriate for the client's level of cognitive ability. In all cases, monitoring clients' task performance and level of engagement informs clinical decision making, such as deciding when a shift in cognitive goals needs to occur.

As task mastery is achieved, the CR therapist should consider adding exercises to the treatment plan to broaden the range of cognitive practice. The client who initially focused on processing speed and attention may begin to incorporate exercises that more specifically target working memory and verbal learning. The client who began with working memory and verbal learning might take on problem solving and reasoning exercises. When adding to the treatment plan, the therapist should again refer to Table 3.1 to consider the types of exercises that are appropriate for the client's learning needs. However, as the client progresses, learning needs may change. The client who initially benefited from tasks with proximal goals may later appreciate a longer-term challenge, and the client who at first preferred a minimalistic learning context may later choose to try tasks with more "bells and whistles."

It remains important to provide opportunities to perform different exercises that require similar skills and strategies. Over time, the therapist should consider pairing exercises that build on one another so that cognitive skills practiced previously will be increasingly employed at the same time. Practicing skills in different exercise contexts promotes generalization of cognitive gains and allows for new applications and reinforcement of previously learned information-processing strategies. Offering choices of cognitive exercises within the treatment plan maintains the autonomy-supportive learning environment and thereby supports the client's intrinsic motivation to learn.

As cognitive goals and exercise choices are adapted over time, learning goals will also shift to meet the client's learning needs. Throughout the course of treatment, the learning goals should reflect the client's progress so as to build on previously learned skills while increasing the level of challenge. Whereas initially the client may have focused on building awareness and engaging in CR, learning goals may evolve to focus on task mastery as the breadth of cognitive practice increases, and they may change further to develop independence as a learner and leader in the CR milieu. Goals that were psychoeducational or insight oriented may be revised to reflect the client's current understanding of how cognitive problems interfere with task performance inside and outside the training sessions.

The therapist and client may begin to identify challenges in sessions or barriers that are affecting academic or job performance or socialization, such as distraction, dysfunctional thoughts or beliefs about one's abilities or performance, and low frustration tolerance. CR sessions can provide a context for helping the client practice strategies to overcome those barriers. As depicted in Figure 3.3, for example, Client A initially focused on increasing her awareness of when distractions occur and what the distracters are. For some, distracters may be internal, such as fatigue, worry, or frustration. For others, distracters may be environmental, such as noise or the behaviors of other people in the learning environment. The next learning goal for Client A may be to identify and practice the strategies that are helpful for maintaining focus and for regaining focus when attention fades. The therapist can help the client discern which behavioral strategies will best address the problems with attention, such as having periodic breaks, challenging thinking errors that interfere with focus, using coping strategies to manage symptoms, or using headphones to filter extraneous stimuli.

Goal setting can also help the CR therapist continue to shape learning behavior with respect to making further improvements in the client's attendance, timeliness, duration of task focus, or level of independence in choosing and starting learning activities. For example, Client A may extend the duration of task focus from 10 minutes to 15 minutes. The learning goal for Client B may shift, with the aim of improving timeliness from 50% to 75% of sessions. Learning goals may also help the client gain confidence as an independent learner. Client B might build on the initial learning goal of identifying exercises that are most engaging and valuable and begin to choose exercise parameters or new exercises that increase the level of cognitive challenge and target new cognitive skills. As awareness, strategy use, and adaptive learning behaviors improve, the client will be more likely to benefit from the cognitive exercises themselves and will develop a set of skills that can then be employed outside the CR context to improve functioning in meaningful ways.

## LINKING COGNITIVE PRACTICE
## TO FUNCTIONAL RECOVERY

During the initial assessment, the CR therapist ascertains each client's goals for recovery; these provide the framework for delineating cognitive goals and placing cognition in a meaningful context. It is important that the link between cognitive practice and everyday behaviors be explicit and be reinforced beyond the initial stages of treatment planning. This means that clients should practice identifying (a) what cognitive skills are being developed during CR, (b) what strategies are being used to perform cognitive tasks, (c) how those skills and strategies may be employed in everyday life, and (d) how improving the ability to carry out those cognitive tasks will facilitate success in achieving meaningful goals. These metacognitive tasks will come more easily to some than to others, which is why this is an important part of CR to practice in each session. This can be done individually, as the therapist provides one-on-one coaching to guide the client's approach to a cognitive task, or in a formal verbal discussion following or separate from structured cognitive practice. Providing each client with a reference copy of the treatment plan (e.g., Figs. 3.3 and 3.4) that links cognitive goals to recovery facilitates these processes.

Raising clients' awareness of cognitive skills, strategies, and their relevance to everyday life can have the effect of increasing the saliency of cognitive practice, thereby increasing the utility value of cognitive exercises. Perceived utility is an important component of intrinsic motivation for learning: People are more likely to initiate, persist, and benefit from learning activities if they are viewed as having inherent value (Choi, Fiszdon, & Medalia, 2010; Wigfield & Eccles, 2000). Actively linking CR to recovery goals also supports the conscious deployment of learned skills outside the CR session. This can occur within the rehabilitation context; for example, cognitive strategies for improving attention (e.g., minimizing distraction, active listening) or improving memory (e.g., taking notes, reviewing session handouts) can be used during other goal-oriented skills interventions to aid acquisition of information. Adaptive strategies can also be employed at home, in school, on the job, or in social situations to improve functioning in meaningful ways.

In addition to linking cognitive practice to recovery within the context of CR, it is important that cognitive goals be incorporated within the individualized recovery plan and discussed with the broader treatment team. By understanding cognitive goals, other treatment providers can gain an appreciation for the role of cognition in everyday life and the added supports they may need to provide in other treatment domains. This is seen in the example of Client B with respect to medication management. The problems with memory and executive functioning may make it difficult for Client B to remember to take the correct pills or to organize and plan to have prescriptions filled in advance. These cognitive deficits also could hamper the client's ability to organize schedules and make appointments, thereby negatively affecting the benefit from other skills interventions being offered (e.g., social skills training, independent living skills training). If the treatment team understands this situation, they can be appropriately supportive and reinforce strategies to ensure cognitive competence to manage the daily tasks. CR treatment planning provides an opportunity to reframe real-world challenges (e.g., missing appointments and medication doses) as cognitive challenges. Clients and providers can then work together to improve cognitive skills, and the client can build a positive identity as a learner as opposed to someone who fails to meet obligations.

When cognitive goals are included within the broader recovery plan, CR becomes an integrated component of a dynamic recovery-oriented treatment process that is shared among the client, the treatment team, and the caregivers. Table 3.2 provides a descriptive list of cognitive goals and their relationship to

*Table 3.2.* COGNITIVE GOALS

| Cognitive Target | Cognitive Goals | Rationale |
|---|---|---|
| Processing Speed | Client will practice responding quickly and accurately to visual and/or auditory stimuli. | Attending to and responding to environmental cues both accurately and quickly is important for all aspects of daily living, school, and work. |
| Selective Attention | Client will practice focusing on task-relevant visual and/or auditory information. Client will identify common distractions and develop strategies to remain focused on the task at hand. | Improving the ability to attend to task-relevant information while filtering irrelevant stimuli is important for focusing on work or school tasks, for effective communication, and for efficiently completing activities of daily living. |
| Divided/ Flexible Attention | Client will practice processing more than one stimulus at a time. Client will practice switching between tasks. | Attending to multiple cues in the environment simultaneously is important for multitasking. Improving flexible attention can help reduce the feeling of being overwhelmed at school, at work, or in social situations in which attention needs to be paid to more than one thing at a time. |
| Sustained Attention | Client will practice staying focused for increasing periods of time. Client will identify strategies to alleviate strain and to refocus attention. | Improving the ability to maintain concentration is necessary to complete lengthy tasks, to study, and to remain alert to important information over time. |
| Working Memory | Client will practice using information held in mind to perform a mental task. Client will develop strategies to help information encoding and mental manipulation. | Improving the ability to hold information accurately in working memory is essential for following instructions, making decisions, and completing immediate tasks. Strategies for improving working memory can be used in everyday life to improve functioning. |
| Verbal Memory | Client will practice learning word lists, verbal instructions, and verbal content in conversation. Client will identify strategies that facilitate verbal learning (e.g., rehearsal, mnemonic devices, chunking) that can be used in everyday life. | Improving the ability to learn and accurately recall verbal information is important for following instructions, remembering task lists, and remembering information essential for work, school, socialization, and activities of daily living. |

*Table 3.2.* CONTINUED

| Cognitive Target | Cognitive Goals | Rationale |
|---|---|---|
| Visual-Spatial Memory | Client will practice memory for visual-spatial information (i.e., location of objects in space). Client will identify strategies to aid learning and recall. | Improving visual-spatial memory helps the client keep track of where important objects are located and can enhance navigation in a school, a workplace, or a residential environment. |
| Reasoning | Client will practice logical reasoning skills to complete simple tasks with short-term goals. | Reasoning skills are important for organizing relevant information and sorting through possible solutions to complete simple tasks with short-term goals. This skill may be used to manage a schedule, travel, overcome small obstacles to goal attainment, and manage time at school or work. |
| Problem Solving | Client will practice reasoning through problems that are complex and carry out tasks that have multiple steps or long-term goals. Client will identify strategies for organizing information, develop a plan, and practice step-wise problem-solving to achieve a goal. | Problem-solving skills are needed to develop a logical plan to complete multistep tasks and to set and achieve long-term goals. Practicing strategies to organize information and following a step-wise procedure for achieving a goal can be used in managing social relationships, living and traveling independently, managing time, and completing tasks for school or work. |

real-world functioning. This information can be appropriately adapted for client records and can be shared with the client and the larger treatment team. For example, Client A, whose recovery goal is communication and socialization, may initially work toward improving processing speed, selective attention, and flexible attention. The corresponding objectives included in the broader recovery plan may succinctly state, "Client A will practice responding quickly to important information needed to complete tasks at hand. Client A will identify sources of distraction and develop strategies for staying focused in conversations to improve communication and social skills." This allows the CR therapist and the client to choose appropriate exercises in session, and it also provides the language for the treatment team to conceptualize how improving processing speed and attention fits with the client's recovery goals.

Verbal presentation of the CR treatment plan to a treatment team offers an opportunity to expand on the written record and describe in greater detail how cognitive and learning goals may be supported and reinforced in the broader rehabilitation context. An example is Client C, who is participating in CR while also receiving supported employment services. The CR therapist may present the treatment plan as follows:

> In an initial assessment of Client C's cognitive ability, he demonstrated poor performance on tests of attention and working memory. From his self-report, his cognitive difficulties may be affecting his job performance at the fast-food restaurant, especially when he is asked to take orders at the drive-thru. In cognitive remediation, our initial cognitive goal will be to practice divided and flexible attention, which entails processing sets of information simultaneously and switching back and forth from one task to another. This pertains to work, as operating the drive-thru requires him to pay attention to and to complete more than one task at a time. We will gradually build in exercises for working memory, which will enable him to practice holding information in mind while carrying out a task. This is relevant to his work goal because he is often required to keep orders in memory while inputting items into the computer. Improving these cognitive abilities may help Client C make progress on his work goal, particularly regarding his desire to take on more responsibilities at the restaurant. However, Client C reported that anxiety has been a consistent barrier. One of the learning goals we will work on will be to increase awareness of anxiety during cognitive exercise. It may be helpful for Client C to work on identifying effective coping skills during his Stress Management group. We can use cognitive remediation as a place to practice managing negative thoughts and emotions so that he can gradually increase the level of cognitive challenge and gain mastery over the skills of attention and working memory. His continued practice of those strategies, here and at work, can be positively reinforced in his other skills groups as well.

By supporting the broader contexts within which cognitive skills and strategies may be used, the CR therapist can play a significant role in helping the client make progress toward his goals for recovery.

## PERSONALIZATION

CR treatment planning is personalized to meet the cognitive needs of each individual. This occurs through the process of dynamic assessment, the formulation of a plan of exercises that suits each individual's cognitive profile and learning needs, and linking of cognitive goals to recovery. The treatment plan should be shared with the client to provide an element of ownership over learning. CR therapists may find it helpful to provide each client with a folder that contains a written copy of the treatment plan listing the broader recovery goals, the associated CR objectives, the target cognitive skills, the learning goals, and the recommended plan of exercises to target the appropriate cognitive skills. A written log of exercises completed and the associated cognitive skills practiced is a helpful tool for many clients, allowing them to concretely evaluate their progress through the treatment plan. Many software programs available for CR allow for individualized accounts to be created; a personalized training plan is then developed by selecting appropriate exercises from a menu of training options. Whether by log or by electronic record, performance progress can be tracked systematically over the course of treatment by both client and therapist, allowing for shared objective assessment of when training on a set of cognitive skills is complete. Before treatment completion, the client and therapist can refer back to the recovery goals listed in the treatment plan and reflect on how cognitive skills and strategies have contributed to the client's progress through the ongoing process of recovery.

## TREATMENT PLANNING FOR SPECIAL CIRCUMSTANCES

When a client manifests challenging behavior, the treatment plan needs to address the barriers that make it difficult for the client to take full advantage of the CR program. The behaviors a client exhibits in session are likely representative of how cognitive challenges are approached in the real world. The person who never wants to try a new task is likely to be rigid and inflexible in other settings as well; the person who has difficulty staying on task in session is likely to experience the same problem at work, in school, and when doing tasks at home. The person whose behavior is emotionally dysregulated in the structured CR environment will likely also have difficulty regulating behavior in less structured settings. These problematic behaviors need to be addressed so that the client can meet the challenge of learning new cognitive skills, and the treatment plan needs to delineate a strategy for addressing them. This section discusses some strategies developed in the Neuropsychological Educational Approach to Remediation (NEAR) model (Medalia et al., 2009) that can be used in treatment planning for such circumstances.

### Rigidity

If a client is resistant to trying new cognitive exercises, increasing flexibility can be incorporated into the learning goals within the treatment plan. For example, an initial learning goal may be to work on at least two different exercises in each session. In working toward this goal, the client may feel encouraged by having a choice of exercises from a selection that the therapist recommends based on the client's cognitive goals. The learning goal can then be adapted, as the client progresses, by increasing the number of exercises the client is expected to try within each session or by prompting the client to try a number of new exercises per week. It is important to ensure that the client will practice cognitive skills in varied contexts to support generalization. Developing a flexible approach to learning also promotes adaptive behavior in other learning contexts.

## Inattention

If a client has difficulty sitting still or too frequently switches tasks, the initial learning goal in the treatment plan may be to increase task persistence to 10 minutes. Subsequently, the goal may be increased in 5-minute increments until task focus is sustained for 30 minutes. By gradually increasing the goal and providing positive reinforcement for meeting the learning goal in each session, the therapist shapes positive learning behavior, improves attention, and more effectively trains the cognitive targets on the treatment plan.

## Disruptive Behavior

Some clients who have difficulty focusing may also engage in behaviors that are disruptive, such as foot or finger tapping. Some clients make comments or noises in response to their learning activity, or even in response to internal stimuli. Such clients may lack awareness of the disruptive behavior itself or may not recognize how much their behavior negatively impacts others. Learning goals in the treatment plan may serve to shape behaviors that contribute to a quiet learning environment.

For example, an initial goal may be to increase awareness of the behavior and to identify when and why it occurs. For some, the antecedent may be anxiety; for others, it may be distractibility; and for other clients, disruptive behavior may be a function of poor inhibitory control. For clients who are responding to internal stimuli, disruptive behavior may indicate a need for medication evaluation, although use of coping skills and therapist redirection can assist the client to stay focused on the learning activity. The therapist may need to point out behaviors that are distracting when they occur in session before the client is able to do this independently. Addressing this issue privately at first and developing a discreet method of communicating in session (e.g., verbal cue, hand signal) may be helpful to the client and avoid undue embarrassment or alienation from the group.

For some clients, improving awareness may be sufficient to reduce the frequency of disruptive behaviors. For many, a learning goal will need to be established, such as developing a coping strategy or practicing an alternative behavior that is less disruptive. Together, the therapist and client set an achievable goal to reduce the disruptive behavior. Workable strategies may include taking periodic breaks to stretch and regain focus, using anxiety management techniques, squeezing a stress ball instead of tapping a foot or finger, or situating oneself in an area with fewer potential distracters. The therapist should reinforce the effective use of coping strategies and take note of prosocial learning behavior so as to improve the quality of the client's and others' learning experiences.

## Reassurance-Seeking Behavior

Clients who constantly ask for assistance or feedback may lack self-esteem and therefore rely on external sources of support to engage or persist in important goal-oriented tasks. This behavior potentially places overwhelming demands on others' time and attention, which, in the CR session, fosters dependence and takes the therapist's time away from helping others. In the treatment plan, an initial learning goal might be to increase independent set-up or use of the cognitive exercises. The therapist would first demonstrate the behavior that is expected and provide adequate scaffolding to help the client achieve that behavior. With repeated practice, therapist support can be withdrawn and the client's achievements noted.

For the client who seeks reassurance and constant recognition of performance accomplishments, the therapist's role is to help the client improve awareness of his or her own accomplishments. The therapist provides support by prompting the client to describe the task approach and use of strategy and to self-evaluate the outcome. Praise should be given judiciously, should be directed toward the client's independent learning behaviors, and should reinforce the client's persistence, independent use of strategies, use of self-evaluation, and task feedback to guide decision making. In this way, the therapist emphasizes the learning process instead of focusing on performance outcome. This approach helps the client develop a sense of competency and increases independent learning.

## Low Frustration Tolerance

Some clients have a difficult time regulating emotion. Given that CR involves practicing skills with which the client has difficulty, frustration and low distress tolerance may present a barrier to cognitive learning. Some clients may act out, and others may give up and walk away. In this situation, an appropriate learning goal might be to draw on learned coping skills so as to be able to stick with the learning activity even when it is challenging to do so. The initial learning goal may be to practice a challenging task, using coping skills to manage emotion, for 5 minutes at a time. The client may even be rewarded for meeting the initial goal by having an option to then choose a different exercise with which the client feels more confident before returning to the challenging task. With repeated practice, the client's performance on the challenging cognitive exercise will improve and the level of distress may lessen. The learning goal should be gradually modified so that the client is able to persist on a challenging task for increasing periods of time. As with the client who seeks excessive reassurance, it may be helpful for the therapist to orient the client toward the learning process and to help the client recognize accomplishments (e.g., choosing an effective task approach) and goal progress (e.g., staying in session instead of walking out). The treatment plan thus provides a supportive structure to promote skill mastery with respect to both cognition and coping skills.

## Fatigue

If a client consistently has difficulty remaining awake or alert during CR, the therapist may need to investigate the underlying cause. Sometimes people have reverse sleep cycles, and with insufficient sleep at night, they are not alert during the day. At other times, significant fatigue is a medication side-effect, and either the dose or the time at which medication is taken can be modified to improve wakefulness. Speaking with the client and other treatment providers helps the therapist determine whether fatigue is a problem in general and whether changing the medication routine is the best course of action. Alternatively, the time at which the client attends CR sessions can be changed if the client is aware that he or she is more alert in the morning or in the afternoon. However, the therapist should also consider that falling asleep during CR may be a sign that the client is disengaged. This would require a reevaluation of the learning activities on the treatment plan so as to ensure that the level of cognitive challenge and the properties of the cognitive exercises are appropriate for the client's cognitive and learning needs. When the client feels motivated for the learning activity, engagement and therefore wakefulness are likely to follow.

The CR treatment plan may also include a learning goal to improve alertness during the session. This may entail specifying sleep hygiene practices to improve wakefulness and likely the use of appropriate strategies in session, such as taking periodic stretching breaks to reduce fatigue. The therapist and client should work together to set a reasonable initial goal, such as to remain alert for 10 minutes before taking a break, and then to increase the goal in 5-minute increments. Over time, less frequent breaks may be required to help the client remain alert for the duration of the CR session.

## CONCLUSION

CR is a unique treatment setting because the therapist is able to closely observe behaviors, both adaptive and maladaptive, that are likely representative of how the client approaches tasks and challenges that arise in the course of everyday life. The CR therapist is well positioned to help the client identify and overcome a variety of barriers that may affect progress toward achievement of recovery goals. The CR treatment plan can therefore be considered an integral component of the recovery process. It provides the supportive structure for helping each client achieve successes in session and in the community.

## REFERENCES

Bowie, C. R., McGurk, S. R., Mausbach, B., Patterson, T. L., & Harvey, P. D. (2012). Combined cognitive remediation and functional skills training for schizophrenia: Effects on cognition, functional competence, and real-world behavior. *American Journal of Psychiatry*, 169(7), 710–718.

Choi, J., Fiszdon, J. M., & Medalia, A. (2010). Expectancy-value theory in persistence of learning effects in schizophrenia: Role of task value and perceived competency. *Schizophrenia Bulletin, 36*(5), 957–965.

Eack, S. M., Hogarty, G. E., Cho, R. Y., Prasad, K. M., Greenwald, D. P., Hogarty, S. S., & Keshavan, M. S. (2010). Neuroprotective effects of cognitive enhancement therapy against gray matter loss in schizophrenia: Results from a 2-year randomized controlled trial. *Archives of General Psychiatry, 67*(7), 674–682.

Griffin, S. L., Mindt, M. R., Rankin, E. J., Ritchie, A. J., & Scott, J. G. (2002). Estimating premorbid intelligence: Comparison of traditional and contemporary methods across the intelligence continuum. *Archives of Clinical Neuropsychology, 17*(5), 497–507.

Hogarty, G. E., & Flesher, S. (1999). Practice principles of cognitive enhancement therapy for schizophrenia. *Schizophrenia Bulletin, 25*, 693–708.

Holdnack, H. A. (2001). *Wechsler Test of Adult Reading: WTAR*. San Antonio, TX: The Psychological Corporation.

Kaneko, Y., & Keshavan, M. (2012). Cognitive remediation in schizophrenia. *Clinical Pharmacological Neuroscience, 10*(3), 125–135.

Medalia, A., & Choi, J. (2009). Cognitive remediation in schizophrenia. *Neuropsychology Review, 19*(3), 353–364.

Medalia, A., Revheim, N., & Herlands, T. (2009). *Cognitive remediation for psychological disorders: Treatments that work*. New York: Oxford University Press.

Merzenich, M. M., Van Vleet, T. M., & Nahum, M. (2014). Brain plasticity-based therapeutics. *Frontiers of Human Neuroscience, 8*, 385.

Ryan, R. M., & Deci, E. L. (2000). Self-determination theory and the facilitation of intrinsic motivation, social development, and well-being. *American Psychologist, 55*, 68–78.

Spaulding, W. D., Sullivan, M., & Poland, J. (2003). *Treatment and rehabilitation of severe mental illness*. New York: Guilford Press.

Wigfield, A., & Eccles, J. S. (2000). Expectancy-value theory of achievement motivation. *Contemporary Educational Psychology, 25*, 68–81.

Wilkinson, G. S., & Robertson, G. J. (2006). *Wide Range Achievement Test 4: Professional manual*. Lutz, FL: Psychological Assessment Resources.

Wykes, T., & Reeder, C. (2005). *Cognitive remediation therapy for schizophrenia: Theory and practice*. London, England: Brunner Routledge.

**4**
—

# Bridging Groups

CHRISTOPHER R. BOWIE AND ALICE MEDALIA ■

## INTRODUCTION

As emphasized throughout this book, the goals of cognitive remediation (CR) are to improve everyday functioning, reduce disability, and improve life satisfaction. To achieve these goals, CR is best considered as a type of behavioral therapy that addresses cognition in the context of the person's life, not just a brain-training experience. There are critical roles that well-trained therapists play in making CR a true therapy. Creating an environment that ensures the generalization of cognitive gains to improvement in real life is one such role.

The therapeutic process that fosters behavior change following cognitive change has been referred to as "bridging" (Medalia, Revheim, & Herlands, 2009). Bridging exercises are therapist-led verbal discussion and skills-training activities that help CR participants apply what has been learned on the restorative exercises to cognitive performance in everyday life. Restorative computer-based exercises are a critical component of CR, but they focus on cognitive skills in relative isolation. In everyday life, cognitive skills are used in a synthetic way. When faced with a task, one simultaneously pays attention to, remembers, actively maintains and manipulates, processes, and organizes information—even for simple tasks such as scheduling a date with a friend. Most of these processes occur automatically, without the need to engage in conscious decisions about how to allocate cognitive resources. Cognitive activity becomes conscious when clients think about their thinking skills and approach cognitive challenges with a systematic strategy. This can facilitate clients' use of newly enhanced cognitive skills while engaging in daily life tasks. Bridging groups literally provide a bridge from the restorative exercises to everyday life; in doing so, they help make CR an activity that improves functional outcome.

*Generalization* is the process of transferring a skill from one setting to another. For example, after practicing a computerized cognitive training exercise, a client applies improved working memory to a real-world task such as doing the mental arithmetic to calculate a tip. It is a basic premise of behavioral therapies that what is learned in the therapeutic setting will be applied, via generalization, outside the therapeutic setting. Yet, generalization does not come readily to many people. In our clinics, at least one third of patients with psychotic disorders improve on certain cognitive tasks but not in the use of cognition in everyday life. Bridging groups were developed to facilitate generalization and speed the transfer of cognitive improvement from the therapeutic setting to everyday life.

## TYPES OF BRIDGING ACTIVITIES

Bridging can take multiple forms. The therapeutic orientation of the therapists, the time available for incorporating explicit attempts to transfer cognition within and throughout group sessions, and the baseline functional skill level of the patient may dictate the choices made. This section reviews three types of bridging activities that could be selected as primary techniques or used in combination.

### Documentation and Linking to Goals

Therapists may encourage participants to consistently document notes as they perform computerized cognitive activation tasks. These notes can be linked to individual functioning goals and reviewed regularly in a group or individual setting to motivate consistent consideration of how to make use of cognitive abilities and cognitive strategies. Form 4.1 includes an example of how a worksheet can be used for linking cognitive activation, strategies, and self-generated bridging ideas.

This type of bridging activity is considered "therapist-light" because there is less emphasis on formulating complex discussions or preparing materials that simulate the real world. This technique also does not require a high proportion of time within the structure of a CR session, although some individuals struggle to formulate their ideas independently and take much longer than others. The tradeoff for this more independent bridging style is that there are challenges in monitoring its fidelity, and there is not much evidence supporting independent establishment of goals, particularly given the challenges people with mental illness have in recognizing and critically evaluating their cognitive and functional abilities (Bowie et al., 2007; Burdick, Endick, & Goldberg, 2005). Additionally, the task can be abstract and may seem unrealistic to participants who are not presently engaged in the types of activities they desire for their future functioning. Therefore, we recommend that this technique be used in combination with one or both of the additional techniques described in this section.

FORM 4.1 LEARNING CENTER SESSION LOG

| Exercises I learned to use | What skills have I practiced? (e.g., Memory, Concentration, Problem Solving, Working Memory, Processing Speed) | How will this help me with everyday living goals? (e.g., Work, Relationships, Leisure, Household Chores) |
|---|---|---|
| *SBTPRO, BRAINHQ, LUMOSITY, other*<br>*Name of exercise:* | | |
| *SBTPRO, BRAINHQ, LUMOSITY, other*<br>*Name of exercise:* | | |
| *SBTPRO, BRAINHQ, LUMOSITY, other*<br>*Name of exercise:* | | |
| *SBTPRO, BRAINHQ, LUMOSITY, other*<br>*Name of exercise:* | | |

## Therapist-Led Verbal Discussions

Group discussions can be used to help participants understand how everyday behaviors are related to the cognitive skills being trained in CR. In this environment, the amount of active facilitation from the therapist depends on the level of functioning of the group and the group dynamics. The capacity of the group members to engage in verbal discussion influences how much structure the therapist needs to provide to maintain the discussion. Even though the participants work in a group setting, this is not a traditional "group therapy" session because of the focus on cognition. The therapist needs to ensure that the individuals in the group remain focused on their relevant goals for cognition and functioning. In a group that has difficulty providing meaningful examples or difficulty keeping the discussion linked to the topic at hand, the therapist may need to provide more consistent examples or redirect the conversation. It may be helpful for the therapist to prepare a number of potential options to fall back on when the group falters. To the extent that it is possible, it is best for the group participants to self-generate those real-life activities that they can link to the cognitive skills.

The therapist should ensure that the bridging activities being discussed are linked to the concrete functional goals for individuals in the group. As discussed in other chapters, goal setting is a critical feature of behavioral therapies; adherence to those objectives set out before treatment provides incentive and increases the chance that individuals will be able to attempt the skills in their own lives. Reference to the strategies that were used to complete cognitive tasks can help participants link their training experience with their real-life behaviors.

The following dialogue is an example of a verbal bridging discussion.

THERAPIST: Now that we have finished our computer training on verbal memory, let's talk about how we can use our memory in our daily lives. On the white board, we have our strategies from the training and our definition of verbal memory. You have your goal sheet in front of you. Who can start by telling us how what we have trained today can be used in their everyday life?

PARTICIPANT A: I can see how what we did today is related to my goal to meet new people and make new friends. I have always had trouble remembering names of people and really anything about them.

THERAPIST: Thank you for sharing—that is a common experience, and we can see how our memory is so important for remembering not just someone's name but things about them that will be important in order for you to have meaningful conversations with them. What did we do today that could help you?

PARTICIPANT A: Well, I need to use my memory better, so that can help.

THERAPIST: What about some of these strategies on our white board. Which could you use help you achieve this goal?

PARTICIPANT A: OK, I could use the one where we repeat the words when they say them and try to keep saying them to ourselves after that.

PARTICIPANT B: Yeah, I like that one too, it worked for me on the computer game, and I have the same problem he has when it comes to meeting people.

THERAPIST: That's great; this sounds like something both of you can write down in your journal to make sure you remember to try this in everyday life. So even though it is not one of your [to Participant B] specific goals, you can see how it can help you in that same area of life. How is it also related to the goals you have in your life?

PARTICIPANT B: Well, at work I always had trouble remembering what I was supposed to do, and like I said before, I just zone out and forget what the boss said to do.

THERAPIST: So that idea of repeating what was said immediately and then again at spaced intervals might work for you too, even though it is a different goal from [Participant A]. Are there other strategies that might work for you?

PARTICIPANT B: Sure, I think they all would help.

THERAPIST: How about visualization; we talked about that one, and you tried to use it on the computer task.

PARTICIPANT B: At work? I guess I could think about what it looks like when the boss says something.

THERAPIST: So, you could get an image of the work tasks you described earlier—of yourself doing the dishes, then taking out the garbage, then coming back to the supervisor to get your new assignment. Do you think there is a time you can try that?

PARTICIPANT B: I will try that again when I go to work next week.

In this example, the therapist attempts to guide the group members so that the general discussion is of a shared topic and strategies but the bridges to everyday life are individualized in a way that links back to personal goals. It takes some finesse by the therapist to help the group collaborate but stay focused on bridging examples that are likely to be motivating and achievable. In addition, the iterative nature of this approach, building on original goals and week-to-week progress, means that the therapist is challenged with preparation and retention of what has been discussed in previous discussions.

Group discussions can be a useful tool for stimulating ideas and helping group cohesion. However, those with cognitive problems may face difficulty trying to retain the verbal discussion and then using it outside of the group. For them, the rehearsal of specific skills during verbal bridging discussions may facilitate generalization to everyday behaviors. Indeed, an active learning environment in which participants are also engaged in a skill-based rehabilitation program (Wykes et al., 2011) or can use role-playing to practice skills (Bowie et al., 2012) promotes greater transfer of cognitive gains to everyday behavior change. This leads to the third option for bridging cognitive improvements to the real world.

## Role-Playing and Simulated Environments

Role-playing and simulated environments are bridging tasks that provide a supervised experience of using cognitive skills as they would be used in real life. For example, in a session focused on encoding and retaining verbal information, the participants might practice recalling the names and interests of people they meet

Box 4.1

## SIMULATION IN A BRIDGING GROUP: AUDITORY ATTENTION

**Listen Up! Improving Auditory Attention**
**Group Objective:** Use auditory attention and challenge participants' memory to answer specific questions about what was heard.

**Clinical Objective:** Have each participant become attuned to his or her auditory processing and apply it a real-world scenario.

**Materials:** Access to Web site—www.storycorps.org. Access the Web site, click on the search button, and enter one of the following titles in the search box: (a) "Claritza Abreu," (b) "Colbert Williams," (c) "Cactus Car Wash" or "Frank Lynch." There are thousands of stories, but it is a good idea to screen the story before you use it in group because some are more discussion provoking than others. Preselect one of these three stories based on which one you think would interest your participants.

*Introduction*
*Today we are going to work on your auditory processing and apply it to a real-world scenario. In order to do this, we are going to listen to a story that someone shared with the Web site Storycorps.org.*

*When you listen to a story, it is helpful to listen to both the details and the gist. By the way, what does that mean—the gist?*

[You can give the following example and discuss it to explain what gist means: *If I said to you, "We went for a walk in the park and it started to look really stormy. I was worried it would rain, so we walked fast. Good thing, because just as we got to the bus stop, the rain started to come down strong." What is the gist of that story?* (e.g., narrow escape from trouble).]

*Now let's listen to the story from the Web site. Listen carefully both to the details and also so you can relay the gist of what was said.*

*Discussion Guide*
- *What was the gist of this story?*
- *Who was involved in the story?*
- *Where or when did the story happen?*
- *What cognitive skills did you use during this exercise?*
- *What exercises are you doing on the computer that make it easier to listen and remember stories?*

*Wrap-up*
Link listening skills to group members' recovery goals (e.g., listening to a friend if the goal is socialization; listening to a boss or teacher).

at a mock party. Box 4.1 provides an example of a simulation exercise involving auditory processing and memory. Some simulation tasks have the advantage of capitalizing on the typically intact ability of patients to learn by doing, a skill called *procedural learning* (Kern, Green, & Wallace, 1997). Whereas many people with mental disorders have difficulty learning by listening because their attention and memory are poor, they do much better when shown how to do something and then given the opportunity to do it themselves.

Procedural learning lends itself well to the concept of bridging and gives the therapist a forum to show—not just *talk* about—cognitive strategies and how restorative computer exercises can assist transfer. Indeed, simulating real-world work environments by creating cost-effective and salient job tasks that are completed immediately after computer exercises produces large effects on cognition, work performance, and reduced work stress (Bowie et al., 2015).

Simulations can realistically replicate real-world environments that cross several domains of functioning, such as social relationships (e.g., remembering information about new people, judging emotions and intentions of others based on characteristics of their speech and behavior), household tasks (e.g., preparing a meal, organizing a pantry), recreation (e.g., planning community activities, navigating transportation), and work activities (e.g., organizing desk space, remembering instructions to complete tasks). Effectively, this technique bridges cognition to everyday life by temporally linking the two and using both to improve metacognition or strategic monitoring (see Chapter 5 for more detail on this set of techniques).

Some—but by no means all—simulation and role-playing groups require more set-up time and have a nominal cost for purchasing or constructing the materials. Additionally, the specific types of props might need to be adjusted to suit the needs of a particular group (e.g., geriatric patients with chronic illness looking to maintain independent living, people who are returning to work after first-episode mental illness). Therefore, therapist demand is higher than for the first two techniques discussed in this section. Role-playing activities also require therapeutic skill to navigate the interpersonal situations that can arise, which is why therapists require specific training in cognition and in running groups with people who have psychiatric disorders. The Boxes in this chapter provide examples of how a simulated environment can be created in a CR group.

## BRIDGING TO FACILITATE GENERALIZATION

Because the goal of bridging groups is to facilitate generalization of cognitive change to behavior change, the content of the groups is intended to address the reasons why people fail to generalize. If one understands what facilitates generalization, it becomes easier to understand the rationale for the various bridging group exercises. There are multiple reasons why people have difficulty generalizing what they learn. Broadly speaking, these reasons can be classified as motivational, cognitive, and emotional. Some groups address one type of barrier—for example, the group may focus on motivation—but other groups address multiple barriers. This section discusses potential barriers to generalization, and solutions, in some detail.

## Motivation and Generalization

Motivation affects virtually all aspects of behavior. It is what causes us to initiate and sustain activity. We are motivated by external rewards such as money or certificates and by internal rewards such as pleasure and interest. In learning situations, *intrinsic* motivation is associated with more learning, longer-lasting learning gains, greater independence in learning, and greater enjoyment of the tasks (Vansteenkiste, Simons, Lens, Sheldon, & Deci, 2004). *Extrinsic* motivation is associated with faster but more ephemeral learning; people quickly learn and just as quickly forget (Schunk & Zimmerman, 2008). Motivation can be shaped by experience and by what happens in one's environment (Deci & Ryan, 2008). The people we interact with also can influence how motivated we are and the types of motivation that determine our learning (Vansteenkiste et al., 2004). If therapists emphasize the inherent rewards associated with learning, clients will want to learn for learning's sake and mastery; on the other hand, therapists who use rewards and punishment will shape clients' expectations that learning is for material gain.

Because intrinsic motivation is associated with greater learning (Schunk & Zimmerman, 2008), it is important to consider what the clinician can do to enhance intrinsic motivation. According to two theories of motivation—Self-Determination Theory and Expectancy-Value Theory (Deci & Ryan, 2008; Wigfield & Eccles, 2002)—intrinsic motivation is enhanced when we expect and achieve success at a task, value it, and experience autonomy and positive relationships while doing it. This means that CR participants will be more motivated to perform tasks if they think they will be competent at them, if they see the tasks as useful for achieving their goals and becoming the type of person they want to be, and if they feel in control of the learning experience and supported by those who surround them while learning.

*What can bridging groups do to address motivation?*

1. As a group exercise, bridging groups are pro-social and can foster an individual's positive identity as a learner with other people who value learning. The sharing of ideas about how to address cognitive health can be supportive, and the excitement one person feels when talking about mastering a task can be infectious. Thus, positive relationships and peer mentoring can make the CR program more valued and more interpersonally gratifying. This, in turn, increases intrinsic motivation to participate in the CR program and, more generally, to use the cognitive skills being taught. In situations in which participants struggle to generate bridging discussions, the therapist needs to model specific and concrete examples that the group can relate to based on their goals and

competencies. Discussing the challenges we all face in making optimal use of our cognitive abilities and problem-solving strategies normalizes the experience and makes participants less apprehensive about sharing their own ideas. Intrinsic motivation can be further enhanced by creating situations in which participants feel competent, because perceived competency is highly predictive of whether people will engage in activities (Choi, Fiszdon, & Medalia, 2010). In these cases, engaging in activities to simulate the real world can create a salient and effective method for bridging. See Box 4.2 for a list of strategies that group leaders can use to enhance motivation.

---

Box 4.2

INSTRUCTIONAL   TECHNIQUES   TO   ENHANCE   MOTIVATION   DURING
BRIDGING GROUPS

Bridging groups are intended to bridge cognitive skills exercised on the computer tasks to everyday tasks. The length of a bridging group can vary according to the scheduling demands of client and provider and the nature of the lesson. Some are designed to be 15 to 20 minutes long and are scheduled after the computer activity. Others are designed to take a whole session (i.e., 45 to 60 minutes). As with every learning exercise, more will be gained from the group if the participants are motivated and engaged. Before starting the group session, think about these questions:

*How can you best reach every person in your bridging group?*

*How can you infuse each participant with a sense of excitement and confidence about using the information and tools learned?*

Instructional style can make a difference in the amount of learning and behavioral change that takes place. Make learning fun. The beginning of a group should be devoted to *engaging* the members; that is, motivating them to improve their cognitive skills. Occasionally, participants are naturally enthusiastic about learning, but more often, they need the group facilitator to inspire, challenge, and stimulate them.

### General Instructional Strategies to Motivate Participants

- Create an atmosphere that is open, friendly, and positive.
- Motivate participants by enhancing their reasons for participating in the group and decreasing their barriers to learning.
  - It is helpful to link participants' cognitive limitations and functional goals to the activities of the group.
- Find out why participants are in the group (the motivators), and take the time to discover their barriers. Use that information to plan motivating strategies.
    - A successful motivating strategy includes showing participants the relationship between doing the activities and a desired or expected outcome.

BOX 4.2 CONTINUED

- Help participants find personal meaning and value in the material.
- Help participants feel that they are valued members of the group.
- Ensure participants' experience of competence by providing opportunities for successful completion of tasks that are neither too easy nor too difficult.
- Give frequent, early, positive feedback that supports participants' beliefs that they can do well.
- Give participants opportunities to have some control over aspects of the learning process by choosing tasks or stating opinions.

There is no single formula for motivating people to learn. When you find a way to motivate participants, they are more likely to make meaningful changes. The successes of participants are part of what will keep you motivated and excited about your role as a group leader—That is what the circle of learning is about. Your instructional style works together with participants' motivations and cognitive abilities to accomplish positive change.

2. Some bridging groups can directly address the topic of motivation and teach people strategies to stay motivated. For example, teaching someone to pair an unpleasurable task with a pleasurable one provides a self-motivating strategy. It is thus possible to teach people techniques to help them stay motivated to do cognitive tasks when they feel unmotivated (Box 4.3). If participants become aware of what motivates and demotivates them, they can self-regulate better.

BOX 4.3

BRIDGING GROUP TO TEACH MOTIVATION ENHANCERS

The 6 P's

**Group Objective:** Introduce the strategy "The 6 P's" to help participants solve problems when motivation is low.

**Clinical Objective:** Help participants utilize strategies to accomplish goal-related tasks.

**Materials:** A handout that lists and describes The 6 P's with colorful images

*Introduction*
*We all have times when we just feel tired or unmotivated, and it is all too tempting to put off tasks until another time. However, as we discussed in relation to procrastination, there are strategies you can use to boost your motivation to start a task and follow it through to completion.*

*(continued)*

BOX 4.3 CONTINUED

*Discussion Guide*
*Let's consider the handout on The 6 P's and talk about ways in which you might use these strategies to help you get things done.* [Prompt participants for an example of each strategy.]

1. **Piggy Backing**: Combine a tedious activity with one that you're already planning to do. [Example: researching new job openings while having your morning coffee]
2. **Pleasurable Pairing**: Combine a tedious activity with one that's fun. [Example: folding laundry while watching television or listening to music]
3. **Partnering**: Have someone do the activity with you or be in the same room as you. [Example: inviting a friend over to talk while you clean your room]
4. **Presents/Rewards**: Plan a reward for when you finish the task or acknowledge the inherent reward in completing the task [Example: taking a break for a snack after completing projects at work]
5. **Pros & Cons**: Clarify your goals to motivate you to pursue a task. What would be the benefits of getting it done? What would be the downside of not getting it done? [Example: Cleaning up will eliminate the clutter around my workspace that is distracting me from my studies; the more cluttered my workspace, the more I procrastinate instead of studying for my test.]
6. **Past Success**: Use your past success as a reference. Can you think back to a time when you completed a difficult task? [Prompt participants for an example. Consider the following: How did you get started? Did you use any of the 6 P's? What were some of the feelings you had after you completed that task?]

*Wrap-up*
*Using all the strategies we've discussed in this group, I hope you are able to stay motivated and continue to make gains as you work toward your goals. If you run into any roadblocks along the way, we can refer back to these sessions to help you problem-solve.*

Thanks to Enid Gertmenian King, CSW, Lieber Recovery and Rehabilitation Clinic, Columbia University Medical Center, for the ideas and format of this group discussion.

---

3. Bridging groups can dispel myths about cognition that might be demotivating. For example, if a participant believes that cognitive capacity is fixed and is not amenable to change by doing restorative exercises, then it is unlikely he or she will be motivated to participate regularly. Bridging groups provide an opportunity to discuss topics that are relevant to cognitive health, such as facts and myths about cognition. This point in the chapter is an excellent place to discuss Carol Dweck's work (1999)

on entity versus incremental beliefs about intelligence. She found that people who believed that intelligence and cognitive functioning was something fixed—an entity that is genetically determined—did not view themselves as having agency and ability to influence cognitive outcome and therefore did not apply effort when faced with cognitive challenge. On the other hand, people who believed that cognitive functioning can change incrementally saw themselves as having agency and ability to influence cognitive outcome by applying effort in the face of challenge. Dweck showed that these beliefs influenced how much effort was applied in learning situations and that education about erroneous beliefs resulted in more effort and motivation to learn. Bridging groups can be used to systematically track success and overtly demonstrate changes in behavior. When bridging techniques are paired with changes in performance level on computerized exercises, the therapist and the group can help individuals view themselves as being able to change their cognitive abilities and change *how they use* those abilities.

4. Many people with mental illness lack confidence to use the cognitive skills they already have or the skills they are developing. Bridging groups that use simulated activities provide a potential platform for demonstrating the existence of current competencies and new ways of approaching tasks that were previously thought to be too challenging. Motivational factors can be considered during role-playing and simulations by selecting those that are most likely to be salient to the individual or group (e.g., talking with job coaches to get a sense of the occupational interests and options available for a group engaged in vocational rehabilitation; dynamic small group exercises for those interested in improving their social relationships). It is also important to match the difficulty level of the task to the individual. Incremental successes are most likely to result if activities are set at a level that is challenging but still within the person's present skill set. This might require some real-time maneuvering by the therapist to introduce or remove elements of the task to match the person's ability.

## Cognition and Generalization

The ability to generalize what is learned in one situation to another situation requires certain cognitive skills, and not everyone has the cognitive capacity to efficiently and easily generalize learning. This is true even when cognitive abilities are the primary target, as might be the case in some forms of CR. Cognitive gains do not manifest immediately, and the ability to put skills into use in complex everyday environments often lags behind cognitive change, particularly if there are not explicit efforts to help people change their behavior (Bowie et al., 2012).

Cognitive barriers to generalization include mental and attentional rigidity, concrete thinking, lack of a framework for understanding cognitive processes (metacognition), and diminished allocation capacity. Mental rigidity means that clients do not move easily from one idea or concept to another. Alternatively, they may have difficulty shifting the focus of their attention. For example, patients may learn during sessions to chunk material on a list-learning exercise (e.g., learning the dairy products on a grocery list first), but when it comes to performing in real life, they might not think to apply this technique to a specific problem-solving exercise (e.g., efficiently shopping by getting all dairy items first). Such patients might need to be taught to chunk in each situation.

Likewise, when someone does not have a framework for understanding cognition, it is harder to activate the appropriate strategies in a given situation. For example, if a patient is unaware that visual scanning is a technique that can be used to capture an entire visual array, he or she will not apply it. Teaching people to think about cognitive strategies can help them apply strategies more efficiently and judiciously. If you teach clients that organization is a way to overcome forgetfulness, then they can start to use organizational skills in situations in which they need help remembering.

Some people have more limited cognitive resources than others, and this also affects how well they spontaneously apply learning from one situation to another. For example, because of limited reasoning abilities, lower-IQ individuals benefit more from training to task than from teaching at an abstract level.

Across mental disorders, perseverative thinking styles can make generalization a challenge. This may manifest in the repetitious use of one strategy that effectively assists in solving a certain set of tasks across a variety of other contexts in which the strategy does not apply. For example, a patient might create a visual barrier to reduce distractions while studying, but limiting one's useful field of view while driving would be ill advised.

*What can bridging groups do to address the cognitive challenges that inhibit generalization?*

1. Some bridging groups can provide metacognitive training; the time can be spent teaching people to think about their thinking. (This is discussed in more detail in Chapter 5.) Participants can learn to be aware that they are using memory, working memory, attention, or processing speed. For example, if there is discussion about using attention when walking on the street, participants become sensitized to become more aware when they are getting cues from the street environment. Instead of being lost in thought, they may realize that they can use their attention on the street and attune to crossing lights, cars, and bicycles.

2. Bridging groups can teach cognitive skills that facilitate generalization. The group format can be used for exercises that promote attention, mental flexibility, and conceptualization. Doing exercises in a group supplements the individual computer exercises, and many people enjoy the pro-social aspect of group learning. Further, some cognitive skills, such as problem solving, are not easily addressed with the quick proximal goal activities that are commonly provided in restorative CR

programs. Box 4.4 provides an example of a group that teaches the use of chunking by time or activity in order to complete tasks; in Box 4.5, a group trains problem solving in the everyday task of meal preparation; Box 4.6 describes a group that helps participants with verbal memory.

---

Box 4.4

## SIMULATION IN A BRIDGING GROUP: CHUNKING

### Chunking by Time and Task

**Group Objective:** Teach the problem-solving process of chunking to encourage a systematic approach to time management and organization.

   **Clinical Objective:** Have each individual work through a problem using the skills of chunking by time or task.

   **Materials:** Whiteboard

*Introduction*

*Many times when we have something we want to do, we do not know where to begin, and then our task never gets done. For example, if I write "look for job" on my to-do list, what do you think my response will be to seeing that? I may not know where to start—and that can be so discouraging that I never start! However, there is a way to make big tasks manageable, and that is called "chunking."*

*Discussion Guide*

*The first question you might ask yourself is, How can I break this task down into chunks? One type of chunk is a group of smaller tasks that can be done all together. For example, if my task is to find a job, one chunk might be to think about what jobs I would like, and another chunk might be to find three places where jobs are listed. After you complete one chunk, you can move onto another when you are ready. Another type of chunk is a specific amount of time. To accomplish a larger goal, you might decide to spend 1 hour each day working on a goal of your choice.*

   Together as a group, come up with a goal such as clean the apartment, pay bills, or apply for jobs. Write the example on the board, and keep track of participants' responses.

- *How would you chunk this task—by task or by time? What would your chunk be?*
- *How does this strategy help you with this task?*
- *Can you think of another task where chunking would be helpful?*
- *What are the cognitive skills you use when you chunk tasks?* (e.g., working memory, categorization)

*Wrap-up*

*Today, you got practice at using chunking to get tasks done. This will make it easier to plan and organize your time in the future.*

---

Box 4.5

## SIMULATION IN A BRIDGING GROUP: PROBLEM SOLVING

### Preparing a Meal

**Format:** In this task, each participant works on his or her own station; the therapist assigned to this simulation explains the task instructions and leads the activity.

#### Materials

There should be one set for each participant, so that all work independently.

1. Pantry with three rows, approximately 2 feet high
2. Empty canned goods (one of each unless noted)—printed images may be used if space or cost is an issue
   a. *Distractor items*: black beans, tuna, Caesar dressing (regular, not dairy-free), mayonnaise, ground cayenne pepper
   b. *Target items*: pasta sauce, milk, basil, oregano, salad dressing
3. Empty boxes and bags (one of each unless noted)
   a. *Distractor Items*: egg carton, curry powder, walnuts
   b. *Target Items*: lasagna, romaine lettuce, bag of mozzarella cheese, spinach, spaghetti, dairy-free pasta sauce, rice
4. Recipe cards with three items each
   a. Original recipes
   b. Alternative recipes
      i. Dairy-free
         1. Spinach salad
         2. Spaghetti (all items available in pantry)
      ii. Distractor (not dairy-free)
         1. Curry tuna on rice (all items available in pantry)
         2. Macaroni and cheese
5. Shopping list and pen
6. Stimulus card with instructions and scenario

*Purpose*

This activity will help participants plan social events and handle unexpected situations while being sensitive to the needs of others. It also requires visual search, attention to detail, and working memory.

*Associated Computerized Cognitive Exercises on SBTPRO.COM (subscription required)*

1. Towers and Basketball: Planning steps ahead
2. Private Eye: Identifying visual targets and ignoring distractors
3. Hurray for Change: Holding sequential information while moving from one task to another

Box 4.5 Continued

*Possible Adaptive Strategies*
1. Examine each item carefully, including ingredients.
2. Move items around to make sure you get a close look and move things out of your way.
3. Flexibly shift and focus your attention among items—the pantry, the shopping list, the recipe cards.
4. Use verbal mediation to keep the recipe items in your mind.

*Related Bridging Situations*
1. Entertaining
2. Household maintenance
3. Staying focused during social situations when your plans are changed
4. Understanding the needs of others
5. Keeping your household or workstation organized so you can efficiently handle tasks when unexpected events make it more challenging

*Procedure*
1. The pantry is set up in an organized manner, with related items grouped together. Recipe cards, shopping list and pen are to the side.
2. The therapist reads the stimulus card, after handing a copy to each participant.
   a. *You have invited three people for dinner tonight.*
   b. *You planned to make lasagna, spinach salad, and brownies.*
   c. *Yesterday you bought all of the necessary ingredients and put them in your pantry.*
   d. *Today, a friend called and asked if he could bring two more friends.*
   e. *One of these new guests is allergic to dairy, so you agree to make a special dish without cheese or milk, and you have time to go to the store and purchase a few more items if you need to.*
   f. *Look at your recipes and pantry to determine how you can still prepare dinner for the guests.*
   g. *You can handle the items and move them around as you wish.*
3. The therapist monitors, takes notes, and encourages participants to handle the items.
4. Participants are likely to finish at different times, so those finishing first should be encouraged to take notes on their strategy and think about how the cognitive skills they are working on are used in the task.

Box 4.6

## Role-Playing in a Bridging Group: Verbal Memory

**"Who Said That?"**

**Format:** This activity is done with four participants and a therapist.

  **Materials:**

1. Therapist key card with list of who said what
2. Response sheets for participants to recall items
3. Self-description role-playing cards with four items that describe the person
   Examples:
   a. Part 1: Where from, where working, favorite movie, siblings. This is all information the participant learned about new colleagues at work with on an orientation day.
      i. I am from Winnipeg, I work at Marco's,[1] my favorite movie is *The Departed*, and I have three sisters.
      ii. I am from Odessa, and I work at the new Delivery Place. My favorite movie is *Escape from Alcatraz*, and I have two dogs and one brother.
      iii. I am from Cambridge, and I work at the Step Up Store. *Casablanca* is my favorite movie, and I have two sisters.
      iv. I am from Buckhorn, and I work at the Stack 'em Up Place. I have three brothers, and my favorite movie is *Jaws*.
   b. Part 2: When arrived, how long staying here, where to next, who with. Here, the participant is at a social event and hoping to keep all of this information in mind to make a decision about which person he or she would like to join.
      i. I got here an hour ago. I am going to leave in a few minutes to go to The Keg with Frank.
      ii. I just got here, but I am going to leave in about 20 minutes to meet Jenny at a coffee shop.
      iii. I have been here about 10 minutes, and I will stay until the end. Then I'm probably just going to check out a movie with Joe.
      iv. I'm leaving now. I have been here for 3 hours, and I want to see a concert with Sammy.

*Purpose*

This task aims to help participants with verbal memory generally but more specifically with source monitoring and associative memory. These processes include recalling not only the content but the context or individuals associated with the content. These memory processes are deeper than strict recall of information

---

1 Fictitious business names are used to minimize associations.

Box 4.6 Continued

and help provide meaning. The task also helps people interact with strangers and attend to their personal histories.

*Associated Cognitive Exercises:*
1. Voice Mail
2. Restaurant
3. Words Where Are You?
4. N-Back
5. Displaced Characters

*Possible Adaptive Strategies*
1. Repetition of material through self-talk or internal cues
2. Spaced practice—recalling what person 1 says after encoding person 2's information
3. Chunking information within content or related to the person
4. Trying to remember specific words instead of the whole passage

*Related Bridging Situations*
1. Meeting new people in situations such as those in the tasks
2. Recalling information about important characters in films, television shows, or books
3. Understanding the needs and backgrounds of others

*Procedure*
1. The therapist breaks participants into groups of four at separate ends of the room and distributes a "Who Said That?" card to each participant from the "work orientation" scene.
2. The therapist has a key card that lists which character each participant is playing and the information each will present. This card helps the therapist guide the recall part of the simulation.
   a. The therapist makes sure participants are aligned in the same layout as the key card and hands out stimulus cards in the right order (i.e., non-random).
   b. If there are fewer than eight group participants, the therapist tries to create an even number in each group and may take on a role to bring the number to a maximum of four in each simulation.
3. Each participant is instructed as follows: "*In this role-play, we are going to pretend that it is our first day at a new job. Here we all are at an orientation session where the goal is to get to know your new co-workers. Each of you will play a role, not yourself. To do that, you each have a card.* [Hand out cards.] *Please read your card carefully, because we will ask you to read that information to introduce yourself. After we have all read our cards, we will see how much we can remember about our new co-workers.*

(continued)

Box 4.6 Continued

4. *OK, let's start with* [person to therapist's right]. *Please read from your card to introduce yourself.*
5. Proceed similarly with all group members.
6. *Great! Now, please hand in your cards to me.*
7. *Now we are going to try to remember some of the information. Make sure you do not influence others. If you are the one I describe, you don't have to say anything.*
8. *For question 1, please think about who said they were from* [therapist chooses a "Where from" item].
9. The therapist then takes the participants through five other items, making sure to not select more than two answers from any one person.
10. *Great! Now let's try something different. On your piece of paper, write down as much information as you can remember about the person to your right.*
11. *Now try to remember as much as you can about yourself! What information did you share? Even though it was not really you!*
12. The therapist leads a strategy discussion: *Remember to look at the strategies we came up with on the computer exercises that are listed here.*
13. The therapist cycles through one or more rounds until the bridging session ends.

*General Tips*
1. Encourage participants to stay in role, even if it does not sound like them.
2. Participants are allowed to read from the cards or try to remember, but the therapist should note whether any divergence is made from the actual card, so that the recall can be conducted accurately.
3. Participants might be reluctant to proffer a response during the recall. This is a judgment call, but the therapist is encouraged to call on those who tend to not provide answers, unless it appears that doing so might damage rapport.
4. Recall should not happen until the therapist makes sure that everyone has had a chance to think of his or her answers.

3. Bridging groups can address the cognitive styles that influence generalization. If someone is an auditory learner and is being taught with visual stimuli, it will make it harder for that person to learn and generalize. If an individual is a night learner who learns best in the evening, morning learning activities will be challenging. When people learn about their cognitive styles and how to use them in different situations, it makes it easier for them to apply their cognitive skills in real-life settings. Most importantly, teaching people that they have their own cognitive style implicitly means that they are learners with style.

That is a positive and empowering message. An example of a group that talks about cognitive styles can be found in the guide to cognitive remediation written by Medalia and colleagues (2009).

## Emotions and Generalization

Emotional functioning can affect how well people make use of their cognitive abilities. We can conceptualize how the emotional-cognitive interface affects generalization in two ways: (a) trait-like attributions and emotional responses to daily tasks and (b) reactivity to specific cues or features of the activities in CR.

Emotional states can positively or negatively influence how much is learned and how one applies learning. The merits of positive, optimistic emotions are easily comprehended: People are receptive to learning when they feel safe, curious, and eager. A bit of negative emotion can also be productive; many people begin to study only when they feel anxious about an impending deadline. However, too much negative emotion can be crippling for learning. Clients who have been traumatized or bullied may feel too anxious to learn in a group environment and may have difficulty finding the confidence to test their generalization. People with anxiety disorders and depressed mood may feel that it is too difficult to learn. When people are very anxious and depressed they may withdraw, and then their cognitive skills do not get used in real-life situations.

*What can bridging groups do to address the emotional challenges that inhibit generalization?*

1. Bridging groups can teach cognitive behavioral therapy skills to address negative thoughts in learning situations. Chapter 7 provides a discussion of how the clinician can engage with the challenge of negative thoughts that might manifest during cognitive activation and in bridging activities.
2. Bridging groups can provide psychoeducation about the link between emotions and cognition. A simple explanation with shared examples from several participants' lives can help the group reattribute the visceral arousal associated with challenge, moving from anxiety to excitement. If the patient is also involved in individual or group therapy for management of emotions, it might help to collaborate with other professionals to reinforce concepts.
3. The use of simulated environments in sessions provides patients with opportunities to directly challenge their negative thoughts about whether and how their cognitive improvements result in generalized behavior change. Simulated environments provide a graded step toward application of cognitive skills in real life. On this continuum, clients may participate first in a memory exercise, then a bridging activity that uses memory in a simulated shopping activity, and finally a real-world shopping experience. People who experience success in role-playing

sessions or simulations have more reason to anticipate success in real life.

4. Bridging groups can provide a discussion that focuses on skill acquisition rather than specific and final outcomes (e.g., milestones such as getting married or finding a job). This can counteract the discouragement experienced when external challenges limit the timing and magnitude of change that is realistic. Patients with mental illness routinely face external barriers that inhibit or prevent generalization of cognitive gains to real and sustained changes in behavior. Patients are likely to face stigma, a reduced social network, and limited financial and personal resources. They often have long histories of disengagement from the very areas to which we hope cognitive improvements will transfer. Change in work requires availability of jobs. Improvements in one's housing situation require money. Socializing requires a network of acquaintances and the skills to navigate complex and ever-evolving social expectations. In discussing change with patients, it is important to reflect on how external barriers might impinge on changes in our domains of functioning, such as marriage, employment, education, and housing status. By focusing on skill acquisition rather than discrete outcomes during the bridging group, the therapist can help to reinforce early and frequent progress in how bridging changes behaviors. Counteracting discouragement by providing a forum and structure for realistic self-appraisals can facilitate the development of cognitive skills.

## SUMMARY

It is evident that bridging groups provide an important supplement to computer-based restorative cognitive training. As their name implies, they are intended to bridge the results of restorative cognitive work to the use of cognition in everyday life. However, they can do more than that, by facilitating motivation to learn and fostering identity as a learner. As a pro-social activity, bridging groups embrace learning as a shared, socially valued activity and teach the compensatory strategies and complex real-world problem-solving skills that translate activation of discrete cognitive skills into a synthetic application of cognition in everyday life.

## REFERENCES

Bowie, C. R., Grossman, M., Gupta, M., Holshausen, K. H., & Best, M. W. (2015). Action-Based Cognitive Remediation for Severe Mental Illness: Tangible Real-World Simulations and Goal Setting Produce Larger and More Durable Effects on Functional and Vocational Outcomes. Manuscript submitted for publication.

Bowie, C. R., McGurk, S. M., Mausbach, B. T., Patterson, T. L., & Harvey, P. D. (2012). Combined cognitive remediation and functional skills training for schizophrenia: effects on cognition, functional competence, and real world behavior. *American Journal of Psychiatry, 169,* 710–718.

Bowie, C. R., Twamley, E. W., Anderson, H., Halpern, B., Patterson, T. L., & Harvey, P. D. (2007). Self-assessment of functional status in schizophrenia. *Journal of Psychiatric Research, 41*(12), 1012–1018.

Burdick, K. E., Endick, C. J., & Goldberg, J. F. (2005). Assessing cognitive deficits in bipolar disorder: Are self-reports valid? *Psychiatry Research, 136*(1), 43–50.

Choi, J., Fiszdon, J. M., & Medalia, A. (2010) Expectancy-value theory in persistence of learning effects in schizophrenia: Role of task value and perceived competency. *Schizophrenia Bulletin, 36,* 957–965.

Deci, E. L., & Ryan, R. M. (2008). Facilitating optimal motivation and psychological well-being across life's domains. *Canadian Psychology/Psychologie Canadienne, 49,* 14–23.

Dweck, C. S. (1999) *Self-theories: Their role in motivation, personality, and development.* Philadelphia, PA: Psychology Press.

Kern, R. S., Green, M. F., & Wallace, C. J. (1997). Declarative and procedural learning in schizophrenia: A test of the integrity of divergent memory systems. *Cognitive Neuropsychiatry, 2*(1), 39–50.

Medalia, A., Revheim, N., & Herlands, T. (2009). *Cognitive remediation for psychological disorders: Treatments that work.* New York: Oxford University Press.

Schunk, D. H., & Zimmerman, B. J. (Eds.) (2008): *Motivation and self-regulated learning: Theory, research, and applications.* Mahwah, NJ: Lawrence Erlbaum Associates.

Vansteenkiste, M., Simons, J., Lens, W. Sheldon, K. M., & Deci, E. L. (2004). Motivating learning, performance, and persistence: The synergistic effects of intrinsic goal contents and autonomy-supportive contexts. *Journal of Personality and Social Psychology, 87,* 246–260.

Wigfield, A., & Eccles, J. S. (Eds.). (2002): *Development of achievement motivation.* San Diego, CA: Academic Press.

Wykes, T., Huddy, V., Cellard, C., McGurk, S. R., & Czobor, P. (2011). A meta-analysis of cognitive remediation for schizophrenia. *American Journal of Psychiatry, 168,* 472–485.

# 5

# A Metacognitive Approach to Cognitive Remediation

## *Why We Need to Attend to It to Produce Functional Outcomes*

**TIL WYKES, ADAM CROWTHER, AND CLARE REEDER** ■

## INTRODUCTION

Individuals with mental health disorders often do not attain their life goals. The purpose of this book is to try to identify why this is so and to suggest ways to improve the quality of life and well-being of these individuals. There are a number of obvious contributing factors to consider at the start of this chapter. Individuals with mental health disorders are often affected by limited life chances. For instance, if the disorder starts early, there is less chance that they have learnt or practiced skills that are important for future achievement, including in the fields of education and friendships. But regardless of when the disorder starts, society also limits opportunities through discrimination and stigma, which prevents the individual from testing or practicing skills. These societal limitations are being addressed by campaigns such as Time to Change in the United Kingdom (Evans-Lacko et al., 2013; Henderson & Thornicroft, 2013).

However, some limitations lie with the individuals themselves and their competence, capability, and confidence in performing the tasks and skills that would enable success in a job or in social relationships. This book concentrates on one area of an individual's makeup—cognition or thinking skills. But this is just one of an interlinked set of factors that need to be addressed in a comprehensive approach to rehabilitation. How these other limiting factors change over time also affects the outcomes of treatment for those with cognitive problems. In our clinical practice, we have often found that change in cognitive performance achieved through therapy actually has effects on those providing both formal and informal support. The change is usually from a pessimistic to a more optimistic outlook, which improves the number of opportunities offered and raises expectations. This means that functional improvements slowly increase over time; often, they are measurable only much later in this improved milieu. However, we have also found the opposite—a falling off of improvements made during therapy when the individual loses access to stimulating opportunities provided during therapy and has less access to places or situations in which to practice and reinforce new skills.

We describe all of this because cognitive remediation to aid functioning takes place within a care system and a society that have an impact on the likelihood of transfer of therapy gains. We will return to this point at the end of the chapter because engagement with a client's social and clinical conditions is vital. An important component of the therapist's role in cognitive training treatments is to support this engagement.

## OUR METACOGNITIVE FOCUS

Over the last 20 years, there has been a revolution in targeting of treatment for cognition in schizophrenia using a new therapy—cognitive remediation (CR)—to improve recovery outcomes. There is now evidence of general CR benefits to cognition irrespective of the method used (Wykes, Huddy, Cellard, McGurk, & Czobor, 2011), but the evidence on functioning is less clear. One meta-analysis suggested that CR that includes explicit strategy teaching and is provided within a comprehensive rehabilitation approach has the largest effects. But this conclusion was based on only a few studies (Wykes et al., 2011). However, it does fit with our own clinical focus and experience, which indicates that engagement with a community that provides opportunities and reinforcement for the transfer of strategies is vital to generalize and maintain therapeutic gains.

When the clinical practice evidence is absent, we can, and should, rely on the well-developed cognitive psychology of learning as well as clinical best practice, backed up as far as possible by sound experimental evidence. A further evolution must occur just to catch up with current learning theory if we are to improve the translation of practiced cognitive skills to other cognitive problems and into everyday life. It is our contention that this means paying attention to two key factors: metacognition and motivation. (Motivation is discussed in more detail in Chapters 4 and 8.) In this chapter, we describe the underlying model and then define the clinical pathway that has the best chance of transferring cognitive gain to functional gain.

## THE BASIC MODEL OF COGNITIVE REMEDIATION

The basis of CR is that if poor cognitive skill is predictive of poor functioning, then improving cognition should improve functioning (Fig. 5.1). Individual cognitive

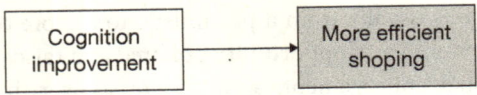

**Figure 5.1** How are cognitive gains related to functioning?

targets for remediation are chosen on the basis of the correlation between functioning and outcome.

However, this cannot be the whole answer because there is evidence that cognitive change in some of the measures that correlate with functioning does not affect functioning and that noncorrelated factors can have an effect (e.g., Reeder, Newton, Frangou, & Wykes, 2004; Reeder, Smedley, Butt, Bogner, & Wykes, 2006). Other data suggest that functional change can be achieved without a noticeable improvement on some cognitive tests despite CR (e.g., Silverstein et al., 2005). Wykes and Huddy (2009) highlighted these problems to provide evidence that CR is complex and that any model needs to examine explicitly the moderating or mediating effects of cognition change in order to provide therapists with a clear set of cognitive targets. It took some time before these potential moderating or mediating effects were tested (as opposed to the direct effects of CR on outcome). In 2012, Wykes et al. showed that there was a relationship between improved work quality and improved executive functioning, but this relationship accounted for only 15% of the variance, leaving 85% still to be explained (Fig. 5.2). We argue that this unexplained variance can be explained by the effects of remediation on metacognition.

It is difficult to tie down which cognitive skill is essential to improvement, although the weight of evidence suggests that executive functioning is the most helpful skill (Eack, Greenwald, Hogarty, & Keshavan, 2010a; Eack et al., 2010b; Penadés et al., 2010; Reeder et al., 2004, 2006, 2014; Wykes et al., 2012). Executive functioning is a type of metacognition (see later definitions) because it regulates other cognitive skills.

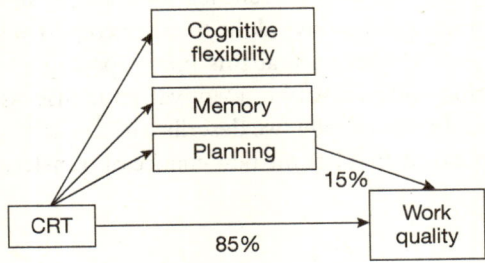

**Figure 5.2** A model of how cognitive remediation moderates functional outcome. CRT = cognitive remediation therapy.
Adapted from Wykes, T., Reeder, C., Huddy, V., Taylor, R., Wood, H., Ghirasim, N., . . . & Landau, S. (2012). Developing models of how cognitive improvements change functioning: Mediation, moderation and moderated mediation. *Schizophrenia Research*, *138*(1), 88–93.

# METACOGNITION AND ITS SIGNIFICANCE IN SCHIZOPHRENIA

The most common description of metacognition is that it is "thinking about thinking." A more formal definition comes from the *Oxford Dictionary of Psychology*, which defines metacognition as "knowledge and beliefs about one's own cognitive processes ... also sometimes applied to the regulation of cognitive functions, including planning, checking, or monitoring." It is not a new concept: Metacognition has been the subject of intellectual pursuit since at least the time of Aristotle in *De Anima* and the *Parva Naturalia*, about 300 years B.C.E.

To be more specific for cognition, the components of metacognition are monitoring (evaluation of cognitive functioning), control or regulation (directing and evaluating cognitive and behavioral performance), and knowledge (understanding task difficulty and the resources required). Awareness of cognitive problems can be thought of as a form of metacognitive knowledge that can effectively guide the deployment of cognitive resources to a specific task and can provide the necessary knowledge for individuals to access the relevant resources so as to perform at maximal efficiency (Flavell, 1979).

Planning how to remember something, checking accuracy on an arithmetic test, and monitoring reading comprehension are forms of metacognition called *metacognitive regulation*. In contrast, *metacognitive knowledge* refers to what an individual knows (e.g., which strategies are most efficient to use in a memory task), including what the individual knows about his or her abilities such as memory. Our argument about the importance of these concepts is as follows: If people want to change their behavior, they need to (a) believe that the behavior can be changed, (b) think about what they find difficult and what can be improved, (c) consider what strategies they can use to improve performance, and (d) put those strategies into practice, monitor them, and evaluate them. All of these components are linked to metacognition and not to basic cognition.

Do people with a diagnosis of schizophrenia have metacognitive deficits, and if so, is this functionally important? The term *metacognition* has been used loosely to mean a number of different things, including the reflection and regulation of interpersonal and intrapersonal factors such as the narrative of one's own life and awareness of symptoms or insight, both of which are problematic in people with a diagnosis of schizophrenia (e.g., Lysaker, Clements, Plascak-Hallberg, Knipscheer, & Wright, 2002; Wiffen & David, 2009). These two aspects of metacognition are known to be important in predicting future functional outcome and particularly symptomatic outcome (e.g., Lysaker et al., 2013), but the focus of this chapter is on metacognition as it relates to cognitive or information processing.

Evidence of a lack of metacognitive knowledge comes from studies reporting a mismatch between individuals' subjective experience of cognitive difficulties and objective cognitive measures—usually in the direction of poor awareness of the severity of cognitive difficulties. However, this poor awareness is influenced (moderated) by self-esteem and negative symptoms. When these two factors are controlled, the awareness of complaints about cognitive problems is aligned with the results of objective cognitive tests (Cella, Swan, Medin, Reeder, & Wykes, 2014). This suggests that improvements in self-esteem and opportunities created by reductions in negative symptoms (e.g., medication, other treatments) might aid metacognition.

Evidence of poor metacognitive regulation comes from the many studies showing difficulties in executive functioning and in the control of decisions (Koren & Harvey, 2006; Koren, Seidman, Goldsmith, & Harvey, 2006). All of these metacognitive problems may be more potent predictors of functioning than cognitive predictors alone (e.g., Hamm et al., 2012; Lysaker et al., 2013; Stratta, Daneluzzo, Riccardi, Bustini, & Rossi, 2009). This is also evidence that everyday tasks and even the costs of care are more likely to improve after improvement on executive tasks (i.e., metacognitive regulation) (Eack et al., 2010a, 2010b; Penadés et al., 2010; Reeder et al., 2004, 2006, 2014; Wykes et al., 2012).

## METACOGNITION, PEDAGOGY, AND IMPLICATIONS FOR THE TRANSFER OF SKILLS

The field of CR, and that of psychological treatment development more generally, have not spent enough time considering both the cognitive psychology of learning and what is known about the transfer of new skills between the learning setting and novel situations—in particular, how metacognition is crucial. We first investigate the literature on learning in general and the more recent research on metacognition.

Contemporary research on learning has concentrated on the issue addressed in this book: How do we promote the transfer of gains made in CR to functional improvement? The arguments in education have been about situated and constructivist learning. Situated learning emphasizes that much of what is learned is specific to the situation in which it is learned and focuses on the context, application, and use of knowledge rather than memorization of isolated facts and accumulation of skills. Transfer is therefore difficult unless the tasks or the learning situation conform to similarity rules.

Constructivism, or problem-based learning, is a method that allows students to learn about a subject by exposing them to multiple problems; students are able to construct their understanding of the subject through their experience of the problems. Constructivist learning is often used as an argument to support specific training "on the job." It has been mirrored within clinical practice in discussions about the benefits of cognitive treatments for functional gains as opposed to simply teaching specific functioning in situ (e.g., how to go shopping). Our argument, which relates to our claim that metacognition is important, is that most everyday problems can be improved with the more efficient, systematic approach. It would be very costly to train on every potential situation, so teaching schema or basic tools may be best. But if the functional outcome is very narrow (e.g., improving performance in putting together a radio), it is probably best to concentrate on the task specifically, because it is unlikely that teaching basic cognitive machinery for the sake of one task will provide benefits that outweigh the costs.

Although these two philosophies (and empirical data) are often pitted against each other, it is clear that there is benefit from both. One of the most famous studies demonstrating this fact was performed by Scholckow and Judd (Judd, 1908, described in Anderson, Reder, & Simon, 1996). Their study involved teaching children to throw darts at an underwater target. One group received an abstract explanation of how light refraction affects the apparent target location and also practiced the task, and the other group just practiced. When the challenge was changed from the practice task in 12 inches of water to a new task in only 4 inches of water, the abstract explanation group did much better. Therefore, abstract knowledge supplemented and enhanced performance after task practice.

General rules about the context of learning from cognitive psychology and pedagogy that might be useful in CR are shown in Box 5.1.

More recently, research has explored the connection between an individual's metacognition and learning and how metacognition can be boosted to support learning. Metacognitive regulation is assumed in the learning literature to be essential for cognitive control in the learning situation (e.g., allocation of study time to different parts of a learning task). Effective monitoring is also essential for self-management of learning (e.g., Tullis & Benjamin, 2011). Evidence comes from studies investigating manipulations that improve monitoring accuracy, which improves both effective allocation of study time between different items and overall recall performance (e.g., Thiede, Anderson, & Therriault, 2003).

Reports suggest that increasing the role of metacognition in learning is cost-effective because it speeds learning. These approaches involve "being aware of one's strengths and weaknesses as a learner, such as by developing self-assessment skills, and being able to set and monitor goals." Another factor is having a repertoire of strategies to choose from or switch to during learning activities (Education Endowment

---

Box 5.1

## General Rules for Providing the Best Context for Learning

- Transfer is enhanced if the trained and generalized tasks are similar in their underlying cognitive elements—a rule noted more than 100 years ago by Thorndike & Woodworth (1901a, 1901b).
- Learning is aided if instruction and training is given on the cues that suggest similarity between tasks (Anderson et al., 1996).
- If knowledge is gained in only a single context, it is unlikely (or less likely) to be used in another context.
- Task representation (whether similar in an abstract form or as a schema) and the amount of practice on the task affect transfer to other tasks, with recognizable abstract forms being more easily transferred (Kotovsky & Fallside, 1989).
- Transfer is enhanced when training involves multiple examples and encourages learners to reflect on the potential for transfer.
- Success in tasks can have differing effects on individuals. In particular, those with fewer skills tend to doubt their ability and believe that success is attained through luck rather than effort (e.g., Weiner, 1974).

Foundation, 2013). A review of meta-analyses of such teaching strategies showed additional progress of 7 to 9 months on average, in pupils' abilities. The effect of this teaching becomes even more apparent when it is applied in small groups (e.g., Dignath, Buettner, & Langfeldt, 2008). Importantly for CR, this approach seems to provide the most benefit to lower-achieving students and older people. One of the key issues stressed in the 2008 review is that it is important to ensure that pupils are not supported too much; they should receive scaffolded learning in which the supports are slowly removed to be sure that learning is self-supported.

The key to metacognition teaching seems to be guiding students by the explicit teaching of strategies for learning and use of knowledge (i.e., transfer to new situations, teaching metacognitive knowledge). Reviews of strategic learning suggest some key principles that are vital in the learning arena; the ones reported here were produced by Simpson and Nist (2000). The principles underlying the ability to transfer or generalize strategy skills from the educational setting to other activities are shown in Box 5.2.

Pedagogy therefore provides some useful guidance as to how we might approach learning in order to maximize transfer. The principles from pedagogical research that are useful to CR transfer are shown in Box 5.3.

---

Box 5.2

PRINCIPLES OF STRATEGIC LEARNING FOR TRANSFER OUTSIDE
EDUCATIONAL SETTINGS

- The learner needs to *understand the task* because it determines the choice of strategy.
- *Beliefs about the task and learning* affect strategy choice.
- *Quality instruction is essential*—learners need intensive and long-lasting training to acquire strategies.
  - *Training also needs to be in three domains—declarative, procedural, and conditional knowledge.* These relate respectively to what the strategy is; how to use it and why, when, and where to use it; and how to evaluate it.
  - *Practice on the strategy in different contexts is important for conditional knowledge* in order to gain the evaluative knowledge of when the strategy can be helpful.
  - *Strategy instruction needs to be explicit and direct to be effective* and therefore cannot rely solely on exposure.
- *Teach a variety of strategies*—including summarizing or elaborating and organizing information. These are not the only strategies, but the literature on what is helpful remains under-researched. We do know that some strategies such as elaboration are generally helpful only for more advanced learners.
- *Focus on metacognitive awareness* so that strategy use is flexible and inefficient strategies can be dropped from the repertoire.

---

Box 5.3

## THE PRINCIPLES OF THE CONTEXT FOR COGNITIVE REMEDIATION

- Both practice and the teaching of abstract principles that can be transferred to new instances of tasks are needed.
- Tasks need to be similar in their components and structures, and these similarities need to be obvious.
- Learning cannot be left to chance, so strategies should be explicitly taught.
- Training needs to take place through multiple examples, which may differ on the surface but build more abstract representations that can be transferred more easily.
- Target metacognition.

## THERAPIST GUIDANCE FOR A METACOGNITIVE APPROACH TO COGNITIVE REMEDIATION

The guidelines that follow are intended to aid therapists with their approach (section 1), their formulation (section 2), their assessment (section 3), and the ending of therapy (section 4). In the first section, we concentrate on the general approach, which can be used even if the actual therapy does not have specific metacognitive elements built in. Therapists can use their skills to help patients participate fully in learning.

## Section 1—The Therapeutic Approach

The following is a detailed discussion of activities that we think are helpful. They are summarized in Table 5.1.

1. TAKE ACCOUNT OF COGNITIVE DIFFICULTIES. Cognitive problems in people with a diagnosis of schizophrenia are pervasive and usually varied, so most CR programs include building skills in planning, control, attention, and memory. Attention problems produce added difficulties for learning, so remediation tasks should be designed to be short and to contain, at least initially, only a few components. This allows the trainee to concentrate on the task with little extraneous or irrelevant information. If tasks are too complex, therapists can reduce complexity by reducing some dimensions. For instance, they can use a piece of paper to cover half the screen, or suggest concentrating on a few elements, or provide some explicit support for some parts of the learning (e.g., remembering some of the items). Only later should the tasks become longer and adjust to changing cognitive ability.

*Table 5.1.* HINTS ON A METACOGNITIVE THERAPEUTIC APPROACH TO COGNITIVE REMEDIATION FOR IMPROVED TRANSFER

| Hint | Process | Metacognitive Development |
|---|---|---|
| Take account of cognitive difficulties | Train multiple cognitive systems. Attention problems are prevalent, so remediation tasks should be short. Therapists should reduce the number of components and remove extraneous information. | *Metacognitive awareness:* The therapist can teach the client to act as his or her own therapist and learn to adapt tasks according to his or her difficulties. |
| Keep success high | Performance should be 80% successful before moving on to more complex levels. High success is important for motivation. Pointing out success as a social reward can be potent. Enquire about success to encourage self-reflection. | *Metacognitive awareness* |
| Use scaffolded learning | Provide learning support early in the program and then reduce it slowly. Point out the learning after the scaffold is removed. | *Metacognitive awareness and regulation* |
| Use similarities in underlying structure between tasks | Use explicit cueing of similarities. Provide clues on similarities between remediation tasks and the real world. | *Metacognitive knowledge and awareness* |
| Teach strategies explicitly | Support self-efficacy. It is essential that learning is not just "by chance," so provide didactic teaching. Encourage evaluation of the usefulness of the strategies. | *Metacognitive knowledge and awareness as well as regulation after the evaluation phase* |
| Ensure that strategies are varied | Use of different strategies, including inefficient ones, allows evaluation of which strategies are useful. Suggest and encourage strategy use. Ask questions to develop self-reflection on usefulness. | *Metacognitive knowledge and awareness and conditional knowledge* (i.e., when, where, how, and why to use strategies) |

2. KEEP SUCCESS HIGH. Individuals with a diagnosis of schizophrenia have problems with motivation (Choi & Medalia, 2010) and have had multiple experiences of failure. Therefore, positive reinforcement should be kept high by ensuring success in a large proportion of the trials. Complexity should be increased only if there is consistent successful performance. The accepted practice (but with little evidence) is that performance should result in an 80% success rate. The background to therapy development is the scientific literature demonstrating that people with a diagnosis of schizophrenia do not remember the behavior that produced success and so are sometimes confused about the right behavior to choose when the success rate is only 50%. Bringing success to a very high level means that there is a clear distinction, and successful (and unsuccessful) behaviors are highlighted. This is sometimes called *errorless learning*. Success is also an integral part of motivating individuals to continue to put in effort and engage in therapy and of building self-esteem and confidence. But success may not be noticed enough through observation of the task or from the computer program's reward system. Individuals can benefit from further social reward from the therapist or from therapist enquiry so that there is some ownership of success. This can also build *metacognitive awareness* by requiring self-reflection.

3. USE SCAFFOLDED LEARNING. High rates of success may be problematic for individuals with poor ability because they sometimes believe that success is the result of chance rather than ability. Therefore, scaffolded learning is needed so that individuals become aware of their responsibility for successful learning. This means that therapists take control of tasks in the early stages and then remove those controls so that the trainee becomes more and more clearly responsible for task success.

4. POINT OUT SIMILARITIES BETWEEN DIFFERENT TASKS WITH SIMILAR UNDERLYING STRUCTURES AND BETWEEN TASKS AND EVERYDAY LIFE. Providing clues about the similarities between tasks practiced in remediation and tasks in the real world is helpful. Even with different tasks, a similar systematic approach may be suitable. Some therapies provide additional support through bridging groups in which individuals discuss how the skills learned in therapy might transfer. Others incorporate transfer by using individuals in the environment (e.g., at work, at home) to support it. Both approaches are clearly useful. However, if the actual skills taught in CR are going to be used in a variety of situations, then it is probably necessary to understand those links during learning. Therapists using a metacognitive approach help the trainee learn the cues that indicate similarities which might prove useful later. For instance, the therapist may highlight how memory strategies can be helpful in an everyday task, after which the individual learns to apply a personalized set of memory strategies in that situation. Transfer occurs through generalization of these strategies to different everyday situations that can be discussed at each therapy session.

5. TEACH STRATEGIES EXPLICITLY. Evidence that people with a diagnosis of schizophrenia benefit from support with strategies comes from a recent study by Akdogan, Izaute, and Bacon (2014). They showed that when learning was self-paced (as in many CR packages), people with a diagnosis of schizophrenia performed much worse than healthy controls. But the gap narrowed or disappeared completely when the participants were given a frame within which to choose an answer, perhaps because this provided a guide to memory search and retrieval. These findings suggest that strategies can support individuals in encoding and recall and, importantly, can increase the success rates within the tasks, thus supporting self-efficacy. Therapists, therefore, should not leave learning strategies to chance; they should provide some didactic teaching and modeling on what might be useful rather than depending on chance learning or on thinking style biases (e.g., continuing to use inefficient strategies). There is now plenty of evidence that use of strategic processing—even if unintentional—by individuals with a diagnosis of schizophrenia produces improvements in recall similar to those produced in the healthy population (e.g., Koh, Kayton, & Berry, 1973). In other words, the failure of memory results from the lack of strategy use.

6. ENSURE THAT STRATEGIES ARE VARIED. The principle of varying strategies follows from the mandate for explicit teaching. The therapist should make sure that the number of strategies varies over time and over tasks. It is important to test different strategies, even if some are not that efficient. Doing so provides further opportunities for building metacognitive knowledge and awareness, particularly self-evaluation and conditional knowledge (i.e., when, where, how, and why to use strategies). The role of the therapist is to suggest and encourage the use of strategies but also to help the individual reflect on when a strategy was useful for one task and not another. Many people find that the most successful strategies are the ones that are already being used, if inefficiently. Successful strategies are likely to be consistent with the individual's cognitive style and strengths.

## Section 2—Formulation

Formulation is a staple for psychological therapies. It requires an understanding of the goals, strengths, and needs of an individual, and this includes an assessment of his or her cognitive ability. Most chapters in this book assume that formulation has been carried out and offer suggestions for assessment. We consider that it is important to include assessments of the following:

- *Cognition*—particularly attention, memory, and executive function
- *Social functioning*—through interactions with the client and discussion with the client's caregiver or service provider

- *Work expectations and experience*
- *Social capital*—who among current contacts does or could the client depend on for support?

This formulation is started at the assessment phase, but it is extended throughout the period of therapy as more information becomes available. It is collaborative and is constructed with input from the client. It informs the cognitive and metacognitive targets for therapy to achieve goals, and when it is shared with the client, it can actually improve metacognitive understanding of strengths and difficulties. The formulation also allows areas of cognitive strength to be reinforced and capitalized on, in addition to highlighting difficulties. Boosting confidence by considering strengths is particularly important for any individual with a long-term condition and much experience of failure.

Formulation is a systematic and coherent integration and interpretation of the findings of a cognitive assessment and should take into account problems identified by the client as goals for therapy. We find that much of the assessment process takes place during observation of patients while they are completing CR tasks. This often allows for a much more fine-grained analysis of behavior and areas of difficulty than is possible with a neuropsychological assessment, which tends to identify only broad areas of strength or difficulty. The therapist must be as creative as possible to ensure that a consistent narrative is developed for the client. Many factors contribute to a formulation, and these can be crucial for the engagement of the client in therapy. Noncognitive factors include motivation, mood, self-esteem, symptoms (in schizophrenia, paranoia is often a problem for engagement), and insight into one's symptoms.

The formulation allows the therapist to test hypotheses about the client's specific impairments in order to refine the narrative and the model. Hypotheses can be tested by observations of the client's behavior with corroborating evidence from performance within remediation and from third party sources. Supporting various skills during a task can also help identify which is the one that is causing difficulty. We find the model shown in Figure 5.3 to be helpful in defining the inter-relationships among factors, and it provides the basis for a reasonable rationalization for the client to take part in therapy.

## GOAL SETTING

The first part of formulation is to discover what the goal for therapy is. The client may have been referred for a reason that is very unclear (e.g., "memory problems"), and unless he or she is aware of the problem and what the therapy can do for a valued goal, therapy may stall. We find that engagement often fails when the goals are not genuinely those of the patient but rather those of the therapist, staff, or relatives. Goals need to be observable problems with a clear cognitive focus, the more specific the better. We call these *Cog-SMART goals*: Cognition-related, Specific, Measurable, Achievable, Relevant, and Time-specific. They are always embedded in real-world activities, so the process of transfer is intrinsic to the

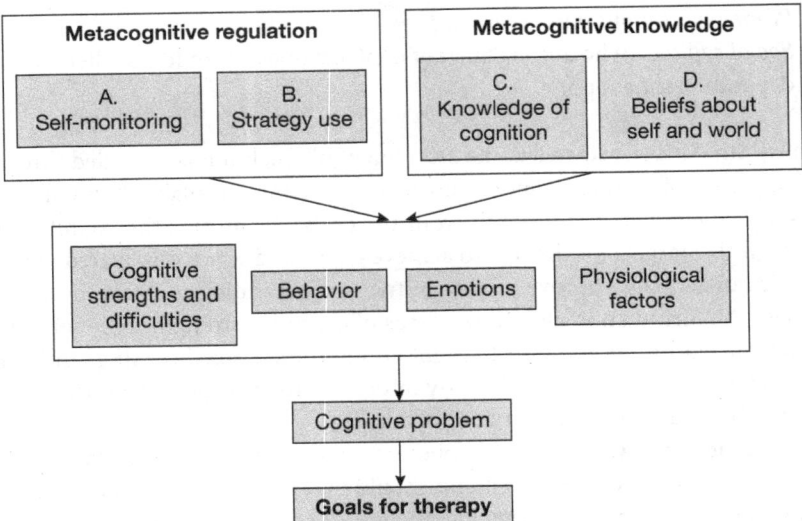

**Figure 5.3** Model for formulation.

targets of therapy. Cog-SMART goals can be formulated as a series of stages to demonstrate that the highly valued end goal is achievable and that it is directly linked to smaller goals set in therapy. Figure 5.4 shows three levels: Level 3 contains the ultimate goal, and Levels 1 and 2 target more specific cognitive goals that are measurable even if they are not tested in therapy.

The decision about the end goal has to be a collaborative venture so that it is cognition related, and this is where the therapist can offer support. The goal (or goals) can change over the course of therapy. Some examples of Level 3 goals are "Being able to remember faces," "Following stories," and "Being better organized."

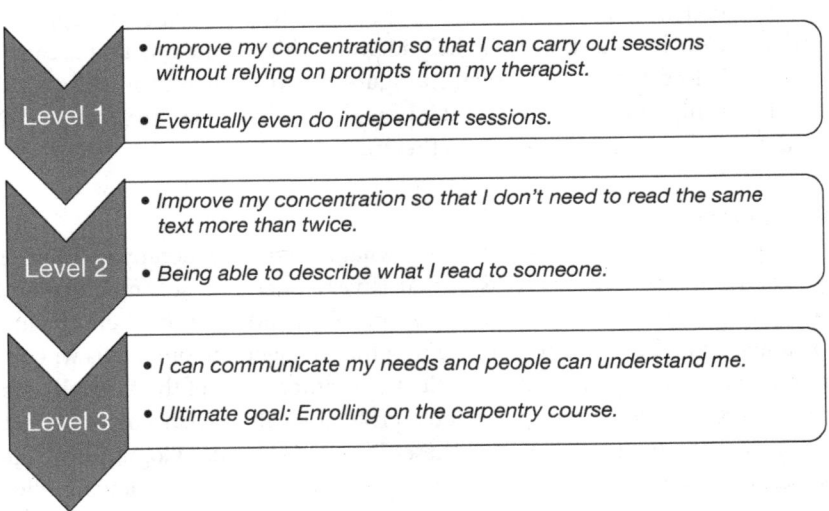

**Figure 5.4** Example of Cog-SMART goals.

## Section 3—Assessment

### METACOGNITIVE REGULATION ASSESSMENT

### A. Self-Monitoring

Self-monitoring is part of metacognitive regulation and is important for a number of reasons. It is essential for making sure that the person is on track to a goal. For instance, he or she may go to the supermarket to pick up washing powder and come back with fish fingers, so somewhere the goal of the activity was lost. This can also happen in the middle of a task, which may be left half done. Self-monitoring is sometimes considered part of the problem for people with a diagnosis of schizophrenia because, instead of recognizing their odd experiences as being just odd, they provide a whole belief system around them. As a result, they do not monitor for information that supports alternative explanations which are more plausible. This lack of monitoring is often what is termed lack of "insight" into their beliefs (i.e., that they are not plausible on the basis of their culture or range of potential explanations). The extent of self-monitoring activity affects the choices of strategies to suggest and the therapeutic process for developing self-monitoring skills. The therapist should evaluate the following points:

- To what extent does the client self-monitor in everyday life?
- Does self-monitoring break down in particular situations?
- What factors contribute to self-monitoring and problems associated with it (i.e., cognition, behavior, emotion, and physiology)?

### B. Strategy Use

Individuals with a diagnosis of schizophrenia tend not to use strategies, particularly in memory tasks in which they need to encode information. This has also been observed for individuals with other diagnoses. Understanding which strategies the client uses and develops is important for the transfer of skills to everyday life. When monitoring strategies, therapists need to capitalize on clients' strengths, such as encouraging the use of more visual than verbal strategies (e.g., imagining the items in the to-be-remembered list, using paper to make notes). However, it is also vital to understand how efficient clients are at using their strategies and to encourage maximal efficiency. For instance, clients may use a visual strategy more often even though it is not effective in helping them to remember.

### METACOGNITIVE KNOWLEDGE ASSESSMENT

### C. Knowledge of Cognition

Two types of metacognitive knowledge are important—knowledge about how one thinks and knowledge about thinking in general. This includes knowledge of strategies for learning or recall that may be known but not used in practice. A list of potential assessments was reviewed by Reeder, Rexhepi-Johansson, and Wykes (2010). Box 5.4 describes some of these along with their strengths and difficulties.

Box 5.4

**Dysexecutive Questionnaire (DEX) of the Behavior Assessment of the Dysexecutive Syndrome**

BADS (Wilson, Alderman, Burgess, Emslie, & Evans, 1996). A 20-item self-report measure of changes in cognitive, behavioral, motivational, and emotional capacity; the final test in the BADS battery.

*Strengths*

- The DEX assesses the most prevalent everyday errors in goal-directed behavior found in those with executive dysfunction (e.g., perseveration, distractibility, planning problems, knowledge-response dissociation).
- It allows calculation of discrepancy between the client's and the informant's perceptions of the client's capabilities.
- Items are easy to understand and are worded in approachable lay terms.

*Difficulties*

- The DEX assumes that the informant's perception of the client's capabilities is more accurate than the client's own, which may not always be the case.
- It does not measure cognitive abilities specifically.
- There is substantial cost to buy the BADS kit and additional sheets.

**Cognitive Failures Questionnaire**

CFQ (Broadbent, Cooper, FitzGerald, & Parkes, 1982). A 25-item self-report measure of the frequency of cognitive failures in perception, memory, and motor function.

*Strengths*

- Questions are highly ecologically valid and are framed in the context of everyday scenarios (e.g., there is a separate subscale for forgetting names).
- High scores on the CFQ are argued to be associated with a true liability to such cognitive slips and not simply with a tendency to claim they happen.
- There is high internal consistency.
- There is good test-retest reliability even after 1 year, perhaps surprisingly for a state measure.
- It is suitable for transdiagnostic use.

*Difficulties*

- The CFQ has questionable construct validity due to disagreement about its factor structure.

Box 5.4 CONTINUED

**Cognitive Confidence (CC) Subscale of the Meta-Cognitions Questionnaire**
MCQ (Cartwright-Hatton & Wells, 1997). A 10-item self-report scale assessing clients' confidence in their memory skills and attentional control.

*Strengths*

- The CC in the MCQ is a detailed assessment of confidence in memory across a range of memory targets (e.g., names, places, actions).
- There is a low correlation among subscales of the MCQ, supporting use of the CC subscale for measurement of a relatively distinct metacognitive domain.
- The CC displays convergent validity (e.g., with CFQ).
- There is significant association between scores on the CC subscale and measures of cognitive flexibility (e.g., inverse correlation with perseveration in the Wisconsin Card Sorting Test);
- There is good test-retest reliability at 5 weeks.

*Difficulties*

- The CC does not assess how confident clients are in their skills in planning, flexibility, or other executive capabilities.
- The CC may be less appropriate for patients with psychosis than for anxious patients (for whom it was originally developed); it has been found not to distinguish between those who are high and low on proneness to hallucination (Morrison, Wells, & Northard, 2000).

**Measure of Insight into Cognition–Self Rated**
MIC-SR (Medalia, Thysen, & Freilich, 2008). A 12-item self-report measure of clients' awareness of frequency of lapses in attention, memory, and problem solving.

*Strengths*

- The MIC-SR assesses awareness of cognitive dysfunction in those specific domains that are known to be impaired in schizophrenia and most strongly associated with functional outcome.
- The response scale—0 (Never), 1 (Once a Week or Less), 2 (Twice a Week), or 3 (Almost Daily)—encourages clients to perceive their cognitive skills in the context of their daily lives throughout the week.
- There is high internal consistency and test-retest reliability.
- The MIC-SR displays discriminant validity, measuring cognitive insight as distinct from clinical insight.
- The MIC-SR is quick and easy to administer.

(*continued*)

Box 5.4 CONTINUED

- Regardless of the order in which they are administered, the MIC-SR may be complemented with the Measure of Insight into Cognition–Clinician Rated (MIC-CR; Medalia & Thysen, 2008), a clinician-rated interview assessing clients' awareness of the same cognitive deficits as those addressed the MIC-SR and to what extent they attribute these deficits to mental illness.

*Difficulties*

- Total score on the MIC-SR has been found not to distinguish patients from healthy controls.
- As with all self-report measures, it invites interpretative bias because clients judge their own functioning.

**Schizophrenia Cognition Rating Scale**
SCoRS (Keefe, Poe, Walker, Kang, & Harvey, 2006). An 18-item interview-based assessment of deficits in attention, memory, problem solving, working memory, language, and motor skills and their impacts on daily functioning.

*Strengths*

- The SCoRS assesses awareness of cognitive dysfunction in specific domains that are known to be impaired in schizophrenia and most strongly associated with functional outcome.
- The questions are ecologically valid and are framed in the context of everyday scenarios (e.g., difficulty following a television program).
- The SCoRS is better able to assess a client's level of self-awareness because of comparison with an informant's responses.
- The total score is strongly correlated with cognitive performance and functional outcome.

*Difficulties*

- The SCoRS requires considerable time and resources because three scores are generated from a 12-minute client interview, a 12-minute informant interview, and an interviewer rating.
- It is reliant on the accuracy of the interviewer's impression and open to bias during interpretation of interviewees' reactions.
- It is designed to be used only for those with a diagnosis of schizophrenia.

**Subjective Scale to Investigate Cognition in Schizophrenia**
SSTICS (Stip, Caron, Renaud, Pampoulova, & Lecomte, 2003). A 21-item self-report measure of the frequency of cognitive problems, with a focus on memory and concentration.

Box 5.4 CONTINUED

*Strengths*

- The SSTICS measures cognitive difficulties associated with schizophrenia specifically, rather than in a broad or approximate way.
- The questions are ecologically valid and are framed in the context of everyday scenarios (e.g., memorizing a shopping list).
- The SSTICS displays convergent validity (e.g., with the Frankfurt-Pamplona Subjective Experiences Scale, or FPSES).
- It displays discriminant validity (e.g., it is not significantly correlated with measures of clinical insight).
- There is good internal consistency for the global score, less so for subscales.
- There is adequate test-retest reliability for the total score.
- The SSTICS is quick and easy to administer (6 minutes).

*Difficulties*

- The SSTICS is designed to be used only for those with a schizophrenia-spectrum diagnosis.

---

Any of these scales needs to be supported by a discussion with the client, perhaps beginning with the results of the scale. Questions about how the client solved a particular task in the neuropsychological test battery would be a useful place to start.

Awareness of one's cognitive strengths and weaknesses and the factors that influence cognitive functioning can have wide-ranging effects on a client's performance. This part of the assessment can also add to remediation by providing some psychoeducation about when problems occur. For instance, the therapist might ask about how difficult it is for the client to remember specific things when he or she has several things to do in a day and is anxious about a hospital visit, or the therapist might ask the client to reflect on whether it is easier to remember something when it is very important.

The therapist also needs to know about clients' awareness of thinking in general. Are they even aware of potential strategies that would help them, for instance, to remember a shopping list? It may be easier for clients to consider which factors may influence other people's thinking (e.g., being anxious, distractions). The answers can often illuminate surprising disparities in what clients do and what they know will help, and this is useful information to develop the therapeutic focus of the remediation (see later discussion for examples).

## D. Beliefs About the Self and the World That Affect Cognition

Beliefs can be out of kilter with actual performance. Individuals can have pessimistic beliefs in their ability and nevertheless perform well, or (more problematically) they may believe they do not have that many difficulties despite clear evidence to the contrary. Explicit monitoring of awareness and beliefs that could interfere with therapy progress may be needed to ensure that they do not lead to a loss of hope but to a better understanding of how to improve. Normalizing examples can help move this conversation forward. Starting with "Most people find that . . ." or "I find that . . ." should help prevent a loss of confidence or loss of engagement with the therapist and therapy.

Beliefs can have both negative and positive impacts on contributing factors to current performance. Beliefs about the self often relate to low self-esteem, and this has an impact on motivation and the experience of reward. Individuals may ascribe positive outcomes to luck rather than to their own efforts, and this can have a negative impact on task engagement. Clients may give up too early when working on a task solution. This is one of the reasons that tasks are provided at a level just within the competence of the individual (i.e., to boost self-esteem). Beliefs about one's abilities can also depend on previous experience, such as at school, at work, or in the family. Belief in a lack of capacity can be reinforced through these routes, especially by the views of others.

All of these components feed into the therapy formulation, which is shared with the client and the clinical team, where appropriate. They also lead to the specific therapy organization, harnessing strengths and developing cognitive weaknesses. Neither can be achieved without some metacognitive awareness. The analysis presented here also feeds into the sorts of strategies that can be encouraged throughout therapy. The final formulation can be set out as shown in Form 5.1 to ensure that all aspects are considered.

## Section 4—Ending Therapy

Even though therapy aims to increase independence through practice in everyday life, the ending of therapy can be difficult. It is important to keep clients informed about when therapy is coming to an end so it is not a surprise. Therapists can use reminders of the ending point, such as counting down the sessions on a calendar. It is important to acknowledge the loss of one relationship and the emotional response to ending the therapy but also to remind clients of their achievements which are attributable to their own work. It is important to plan how skills will be maintained and improved. Follow-up sessions might be included so that the ending is less abrupt and to help with maintenance. However, it is also important to emphasize that even if specific tasks on the computer are not being practiced as frequently, the cognitive and metacognitive skills will be practiced every day.

| Metacognitive CRT FORMULATION | |
|---|---|
| **Name** | **Age (in years and months)** |
| | |
| **Education** | |
| | |
| **Current and previous employment** | |
| | |
| **Current and previous interests** | |
| | |
| **Cognitive function** | |

| Difficulties | Strengths |
|---|---|
| 1. | 1. |
| 2. | 2. |
| 3. | 3. |

| **Noncognitive factors** | |
|---|---|
| Emotional<br>Behavioral<br>Physiological<br>*Consider coping strategies* | |

| Difficulties | Strengths |
|---|---|
| 1. | 1. |
| 2. | 2. |
| 3. | 3. |

| **Metacognition** | |
|---|---|
| Self-monitoring (of cognition and factors affecting cognition) | |

| Difficulties | Strengths |
|---|---|
| 1. | 1. |
| 2. | 2. |
| 3. | 3. |

| Strategies | |
|---|---|
| Helpful<br>1.<br>2.<br>3. | Unhelpful<br>1.<br>2.<br>3. |
| Metacognitive knowledge and beliefs about cognition in general | |
| Helpful<br>1.<br>2.<br>3. | Unhelpful<br>1.<br>2.<br>3. |
| Metacognitive knowledge and beliefs about self (in relation to own cognition and factors such as self-efficacy that affect cognition) | |
| Helpful<br>1.<br>2.<br>3. | Unhelpful<br>1.<br>2.<br>3. |
| **Problems**<br>1.<br>2.<br>3. | **CoG-SMART Goals**<br>1.<br>2.<br>3. |

# EMBEDDING METACOGNITION IN THERAPY: COMPUTERIZED INTERACTIVE REMEDIATION OF COGNITION AND THINKING SKILLS

Our current CR software—Computerized Interactive Remediation of Cognition and Thinking Skills, or CIRCuiTS—brings together (a) existing knowledge of best practices to promote cognitive and functional change in clinical and nonclinical populations and (b) feasibility of implementation, particularly by enhancing acceptability to users. It is ambitious in fostering the transfer of new cognitive skills to everyday life within the program itself, rather than relying on bridging sessions or adjunctive rehabilitation. This is underpinned by the model we have described here. This suggests that cognitive skills will be used to benefit everyday functioning only if two factors are in place. The first is metacognitive knowledge about one's own strengths and difficulties and how thinking skills and strategies can affect behavior in general. The second is metacognitive regulation of one's own behavior. Both are needed to guide the adoption of new behaviors (Wykes & Reeder, 2005).

CIRCuiTS emphasizes the conditions for transfer within the therapy by presenting tasks in the context of virtual situations such as shopping or cooking. But we also use the individual's social milieu to support transfer, and the therapist (as well as the computer program) cues the potential uses of different strategies and the underlying similarities between tasks and everyday life. Both of these approaches support metacognitive awareness and knowledge and increase the potential for metacognitive regulation.

From the beginning of our development process, we involved both service users with a diagnosis of schizophrenia and CR therapists so that we had a program that was acceptable to all. First, we wanted to provide a context for learning, so the program activities are based around a virtual "village," and the tasks and exercises take place in relevant buildings.

The development of metacognition is explicitly targeted through a "metacognitive journey," which emphasizes the reasons for therapy, how personal goals might be met, the development of metacognition and the transfer process, and monitoring of achievements. It includes the client's Cog-SMART real-world goals and the strategies that can be used in real-world situations to achieve those goals. This is all held in a client-accessible library that shows the scores on tasks and gives hints as to what potential tasks or strategies might be tried next. These stages are intended to be used flexibly and to be revisited throughout the program. Figure 5.5 shows two of the screens on strategies.

In order to improve metacognitive regulation, we aim to teach people to adopt a systematic approach so that, in carrying out each task, there is (a) a period of understanding what is required and how task performance is likely to be affected by one's cognitive strengths and difficulties, then planning one's approach to the task (including the use of strategies); (b) implementation of the plans and strategies, which are carefully monitored for success; and (c) review, which allows for

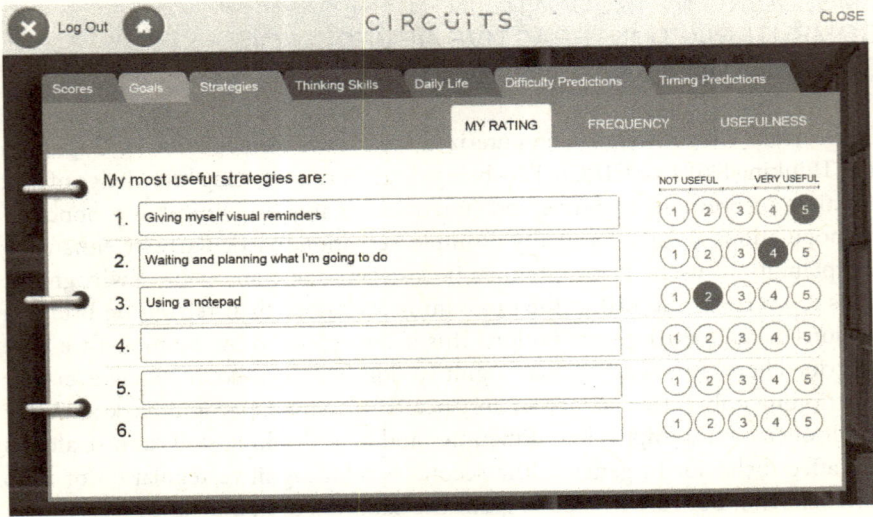

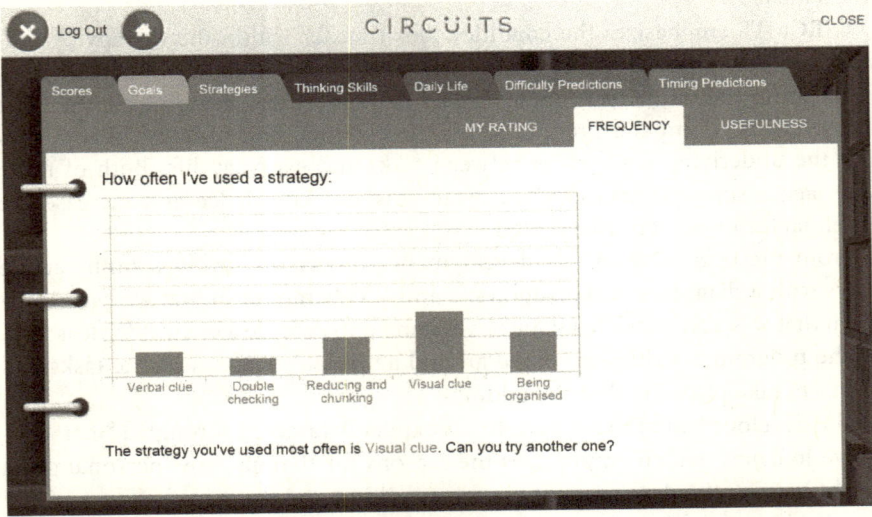

**Figure 5.5** Screenshots for monitoring strategy use in CIRCuiTS.

both error correction and learning by experience. We ensure that these stages are considered because the program demands that clients rate the anticipated task difficulty, estimate how long it will take, and identify strategies they will use to complete the task. Figure 5.6 shows an example.

After the task, metacognitive reflection is required. Clients see their score and rate how difficult the task actually was and how useful their strategies were. This process allows individuals to "think ahead" but also to reflect on their progress,

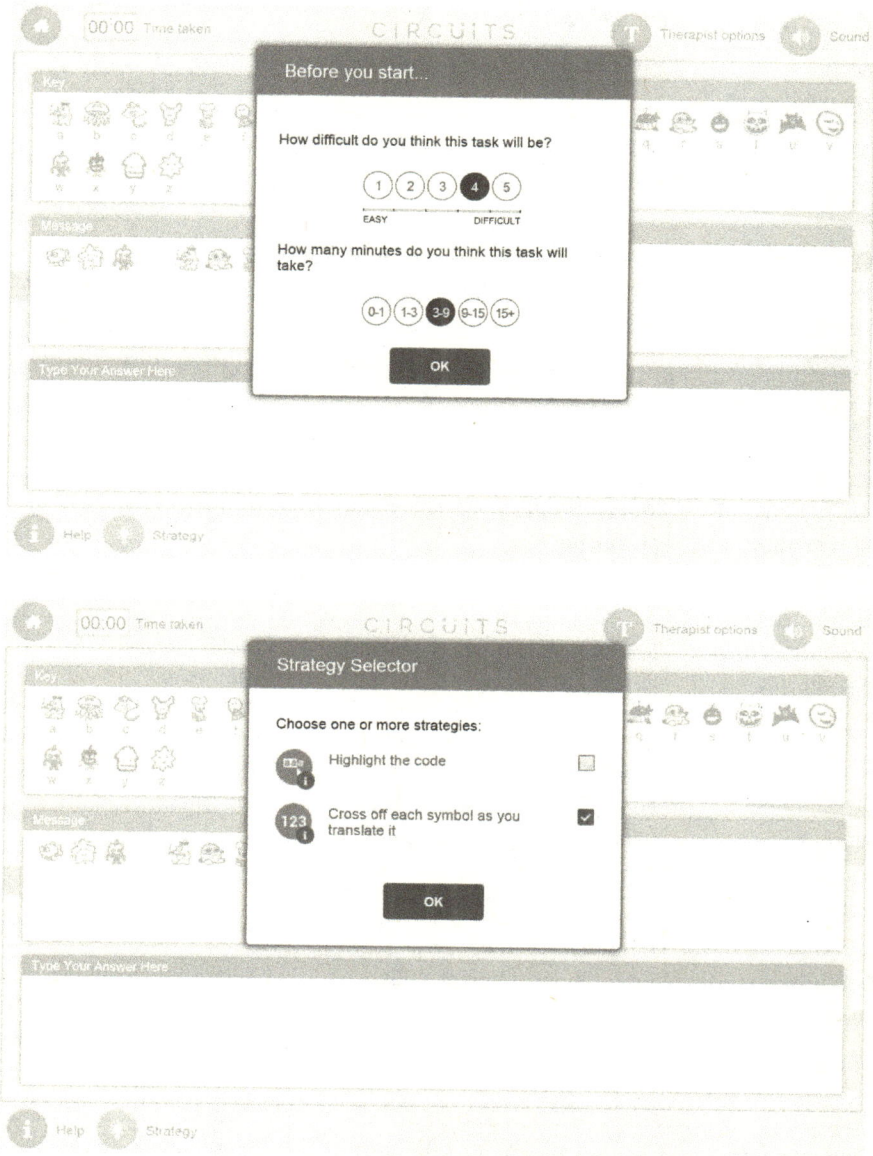

**Figure 5.6** Screenshots for task difficulty and length ratings in CIRCuiTS.

thus encouraging the development of metacognitive knowledge. Table 5.2 summarizes the specific components of the CIRCuiTS program and how each contributes to metacognitive development and transfer.

*Table 5.2.* OVERVIEW OF CIRCUITS

| Specific Component | Why Used | Metacognitive and Transfer Effects |
|---|---|---|
| Short tasks | Overcomes attention problems | *Increases likelihood of success* *Improves self-esteem and self-efficacy* |
| Few stimuli included in a task | Prevents attention to irrelevant detail | *Increases focus on specific important cues* |
| High success rates | Increases reinforcement Improves confidence Increases engagement with tasks | *Increases success, self-esteem and self-efficacy* |
| Few cognitive skills required initially | Trains specific aspects of cognitive processing Highlights specific strengths and weaknesses | *Increases cognitive focus* *Builds metacognitive awareness* |
| Explicit teaching of strategies | Removes the hit-or-miss aspect of learning strategies Allows a list of different strategies to be evaluated (not all will be helpful) Follows pedagogical advice about the need to highlight important aspects of tasks, especially when they might be missed by a novice learner | *Builds metacognitive knowledge* *Builds metacognitive regulation* *Builds metacognitive awareness* |
| Multiple cognitive tasks | Trains many different skills, which can then be embedded in complex tasks Allows use of expert skills to supplement areas of weakness | *Builds metacognitive knowledge* *Builds metacognitive awareness* |
| Content neutral | Focuses attention on the abstract form and cognitive operations | *Builds schema representation* *Increases automatization* |
| Exercises like real-life tasks | Provides a clear focus from within the program to everyday life | *Increases transfer* by embedding operations in ecologically relevant tasks |

*Table 5.2* CONTINUED

| Specific Component | Why Used | Metacognitive and Transfer Effects |
|---|---|---|
| METACOGNITIVE JOURNEY | | |
| Goals | Increases motivation and engagement Collaborative development of goals is part of therapeutic engagement | *Increases metacognitive awareness* |
| Formulation and assessment | Starts at the beginning of therapy to drive the initial focus on skills and strategy development Collaborative method allows for engagement | *Increases metacognitive awareness* |
| Setting the parameters of the task (e.g., how long it will take) | Initial and follow-up parameters allow reflection on the differences between them and focus attention on inappropriate self-awareness (i.e., metacognition) | *Increases metacognitive awareness* *Builds metacognitive knowledge (e.g., by assessing strategies and how they help or don't help with task performance)* |
| Hints for the use of different strategies | Provides time to reflect on the strategies and how they might be used as well as the program itself | *Increases metacognitive awareness* |
| Hints about everyday life | Enables transfer of strategies into everyday life | *Increases transfer* *Builds metacognitive awareness* |
| Homework | Along with therapist-supported sessions, promotes skill transfer and generates confidence in independent skill use | *Increases transfer* *Builds metacognition* |

## CONCLUSION

A final, important point, which was introduced at the start of this chapter, is that throughout therapy there should be engagement with social and work environments in order to aid transfer. Even after therapy has ended, encouraging ongoing involvement within a varied community setting is vital if clients are to continue to practice and develop their new thinking skills in a number of different contexts. These supports can provide a link for maintaining gains after the end of therapy by aiding the generalization and transfer of cognitive skills in clients' everyday lives. We cannot predict whether an individual will need booster sessions to maintain gains, nor how many or when, and this may depend on the types of behavior exhibited by the client. Further investigation and data are needed to support the delivery of a therapy that can reliably boost recovery, especially in those who have often failed in rehabilitation programs in the past.

## REFERENCES

Akdogan, E., Izaute, M., & Bacon, E. (2014). Preserved strategic grain-size regulation in memory reporting in patients with schizophrenia. *Biological Psychiatry, 76*(2), 154–159.

Anderson, J. R., Reder, L. M., & Simon, H. A. (1996). Situated learning and education. *Educational Researcher, 25*(4), 5–11.

Broadbent, D. E., Cooper, P. F., FitzGerald, P., & Parkes, K. R. (1982). The cognitive failures questionnaire (CFQ) and its correlates. *British Journal of Clinical Psychology, 21*(1), 1–16.

Cartwright-Hatton, S., & Wells, A. (1997). Beliefs about worry and intrusions: The Meta-Cognitions Questionnaire and its correlates. *Journal of Anxiety Disorders, 11*(3), 279–296.

Cella, M., Swan, S., Medin, E., Reeder, C., & Wykes, T. (2014). Metacognitive awareness of cognitive problems in schizophrenia: Exploring the role of symptoms and self-esteem. *Psychological Medicine, 44*(3), 469–476.

Choi, J., & Medalia, A. (2010). Intrinsic motivation and learning in a schizophrenia spectrum sample. *Schizophrenia Research, 118*(1–3), 12–19.

Dignath, C., Buettner, G., & Langfeldt, H. P. (2008). How can primary school students learn self-regulated learning strategies most effectively? A meta-analysis on self-regulation training programmes. *Educational Research Review, 3*(2), 101–129.

Eack, S. M., Greenwald, D. P., Hogarty, S. S., & Keshavan, M. S. (2010a). One-year durability of the effects of cognitive enhancement therapy on functional outcome in early schizophrenia. *Schizophrenia Research, 120*(1–3), 210–216.

Eack, S. M., Hogarty, G. E., Cho, R. Y., Prasad, K. M. R., Greenwald, D. P., Hogarty, S. S., & Keshavan, M. S. (2010b). Neuroprotective effects of cognitive enhancement therapy against gray matter loss in early schizophrenia: Results from a 2-year randomized controlled trial. *Archives of General Psychiatry, 67*(7), 674–682.

Education Endowment Foundation. (2015). *Meta-cognition and self-regulation.* Retrieved from https://educationendowmentfoundation.org.uk/toolkit/toolkit-a-z/meta-cognitive-and-self-regulation-strategies/

Evans-Lacko, S., Malcolm, E., West, K., Rose, D., London, J., Rüsch, N., . . . & Thornicroft, G. (2013). Influence of Time to Change's social marketing interventions on stigma in England 2009–2011. *British Journal of Psychiatry, 202*(suppl. 55), s77–s88.

Flavell, J. H. (1979). Metacognition and cognitive monitoring: A new area of cognitive-developmental inquiry. *American Psychologist, 34*(10), 906–911.

Hamm, J. A., Renard, S. B., Fogley, R. L., Leonhardt, B. L., Dimaggio, G., Buck, K. D., & Lysaker, P. H. (2012). Metacognition and social cognition in schizophrenia: Stability and relationship to concurrent and prospective symptom assessments. *Journal of Clinical Psychology, 68*(12), 1303–1312.

Henderson, C., & Thornicroft, G. (2013). Evaluation of the Time to Change programme in England 2008–2011. *British Journal of Psychiatry, 202*(suppl. 55), s45–s48.

Judd, C. H. (1908). The relation of special training to general intelligence. *Educational Review, 36,* 28–42.

Keefe, R. S. E., Poe, M., Walker, T. M., Kang, J. W., & Harvey, P. D. (2006). The schizophrenia cognition rating scale: An interview-based assessment and its relationship to cognition, real-world functioning, and functional capacity. *American Journal of Psychiatry, 163*(3), 426–432.

Koh, S. D., Kayton, L., & Berry, R. (1973). Mnemonic organization in young nonpsychotic schizophrenics. *Journal of Abnormal Psychology, 81*(3), 299–310.

Koren, D., & Harvey, P. D. (2006). Closing the gap between cognitive performance and real-world functional outcome in schizophrenia: The importance of metacognition. *Current Psychiatry Reviews, 2*(2), 189–198.

Koren, D., Seidman, L. J., Goldsmith, M., & Harvey, P. D. (2006). Real-world cognitive—and metacognitive—dysfunction in schizophrenia: A new approach for measuring (and remediating) more "right stuff." *Schizophrenia Bulletin, 32*(2), 310–326.

Kotovsky, K., & Fallside, D. (1989). Representation and transfer in problem solving. In D. Klahr & K. Kotovsky (Eds.), *Complex information processing: The impact of Herbert A. Simon* (pp. 69–108). Hixllsdale, NJ: Erlbaum.

Lysaker, P. H., Clements, C. A., Plascak-Hallberg, C. D., Knipscheer, S. J., & Wright, D. E. (2002). Insight and personal narratives of illness in schizophrenia. *Psychiatry, 65*(3), 197–206.

Lysaker, P. H., Gumley, A., Luedtke, B., Buck, K. D., Ringer, J. M., Olesek, K., . . . & Dimaggio, G. (2013). Social cognition and metacognition in schizophrenia: Evidence of their independence and linkage with outcomes. *Acta Psychiatrica Scandinavica, 127*(3), 239–247.

Medalia, A., & Thysen, J. (2008). Insight into neurocognitive dysfunction in schizophrenia. *Schizophrenia Bulletin, 34*(6), 1221–1230.

Medalia, A., Thysen, J., & Freilich, B. (2008). Do people with schizophrenia who have objective cognitive impairment identify cognitive deficits on a self report measure? *Schizophrenia Research, 105*(1–3), 156–164.

Morrison, A. P., Wells, A., & Nothard, S. (2000). Cognitive factors in predisposition to auditory and visual hallucinations. *British Journal of Clinical Psychology, 39*(1), 67–78.

Penadés, R., Catalán R., Puig, Ol, Masana, G., Pujol, N., Navarro, V., Guarch, J., & Gastó, C. (2010) Executive function needs to be targeted to improve social functioning with Cognitive Remediation Therapy (CRT) in schizophrenia. *Psychiatry Research, 177,* 41–45.

Reeder, C., Harris, V., Pickles, A., Patel, A., Cella, M., & Wykes, T. (2014). Does change in cognitive function predict change in costs of care for people with a schizophrenia diagnosis following cognitive remediation therapy? *Schizophrenia Bulletin, 40*(6), 1472–1481.

Reeder, C., Newton, E., Frangou, S., & Wykes, T. (2004). Which executive skills should we target to affect social functioning and symptom change? A study of a cognitive remediation therapy program. *Schizophrenia Bulletin, 30*(1), 87–100.

Reeder, C., Rexhepi-Johansson, T., & Wykes, T. (2010). Different components of metacognition and their relationship to psychotic-like experiences. *Behavioural and Cognitive Psychotherapy, 38*(1), 49–57.

Reeder, C., Smedley, N., Butt, K., Bogner, D., & Wykes, T. (2006). Cognitive predictors of social functioning improvements following cognitive remediation for schizophrenia. *Schizophrenia Bulletin, 32*(suppl. 1), S123–S131.

Silverstein, S. M., Hatashita-Wong, M., Solak, B. A., Uhlhaas, P., Landa, Y., Wilkniss, S. M., . . . & Smith, T. E. (2005). Effectiveness of a two-phase cognitive rehabilitation intervention for severely impaired schizophrenia patients. *Psychological Medicine*, 35(6), 829–837.

Simpson, M. L., & Nist, S. L. (2000). An update on strategic learning: It's more than textbook reading strategies. *Journal of Adolescent and Adult Literacy*, 43(6), 528–541.

Stip, E., Caron, J., Renaud, S., Pampoulova, T., & Lecomte, Y. (2003). Exploring cognitive complaints in schizophrenia: The Subjective Scale to Investigate Cognition in Schizophrenia. *Comprehensive Psychiatry*, 44(4), 331–340.

Stratta, P., Daneluzzo, E., Riccardi, I., Bustini, M., & Rossi, A. (2009). Metacognitive ability and social functioning are related in persons with schizophrenic disorder. *Schizophrenia Research*, 108(1–3), 301–302.

Thiede, K. W., Anderson, M. C. M., & Therriault, D. (2003). Accuracy of metacognitive monitoring affects learning of texts. *Journal of Educational Psychology*, 95(1), 66–73.

Thorndike, E. L., & Woodworth, R. S. (1901a). The influence of improvement in one mental function upon the efficiency of other functions: II. The estimation of magnitudes. *Psychological Review*, 8(4), 384–395.

Thorndike, E. L., & Woodworth, R. S. (1901b). The influence of improvement in one mental function upon the efficiency of other functions: Functions involving attention, observation and discrimination. *Psychological Review*, 8(6), 553–564.

Tullis, J. G., & Benjamin, A. S. (2011). On the effectiveness of self-paced learning. *Journal of Memory and Language*, 64(2), 109–118.

Weiner, B. (1974). *Achievement motivation and attribution theory*. Morristown, NJ: General Learning Press.

Wiffen, B., & David, A. (2009) Metacognition, mindreading, and insight in schizophrenia. *Behavioral and Brain Sciences*, 32, 161–162.

Wilson, B. A., Alderman, N., Burgess, P. W., Emslie, H., & Evans, J. J. (1996). *Behavioural assessment of the dysexecutive syndrome*. St. Edmunds, UK: Thames Valley Test Company.

Wykes, T., & Huddy, V. (2009). Cognitive remediation for schizophrenia: It is even more complicated. *Current Opinion in Psychiatry*, 22(2), 161–167.

Wykes, T., Huddy, V., Cellard, C., McGurk, S. R., & Czobor, P. (2011). A meta-analysis of cognitive remediation for schizophrenia: Methodology and effect sizes. *American Journal of Psychiatry*, 168(5), 472–485.

Wykes, T., & Reeder, C. (2005). *Cognitive remediation therapy for schizophrenia: Theory and practice*. London, UK: Brunner Routledge.

Wykes, T., Reeder, C., Huddy, V., Taylor, R., Wood, H., Ghirasim, N., . . . & Landau, S. (2012). Developing models of how cognitive improvements change functioning: Mediation, moderation and moderated mediation. *Schizophrenia Research*, 138(1), 88–93.

# 6

# Implementation and Dissemination of Evidenced-Based Mental Health Practices

**FRANCES DARK** ■

## INTRODUCTION

There is a global consensus that improving health care outcomes requires the routine use of evidenced-based care. Realizing this goal has been problematic, not least because it involves a change in clinician behavior, and implementation research, which might illuminate how best to achieve this change, is relatively immature compared to efficacy and effectiveness research. The latter studies identify interventions with evidence of scientific rigor from randomized controlled trials and meta-analyses. Implementation research champions external, ecological validity. How do evidence-based interventions perform in the "real world" when applied to diverse populations and diverse contexts?

This chapter aims to provide a guide to the systematic implementation and dissemination of cognitive remediation (CR) programs into mental health care. Mental health services (MHSs) are heterogeneous, with variations between districts and regions as well as globally. Frameworks to facilitate implementation in diverse settings while retaining the core effective components of CR are presented. The evidence for CR comes predominantly from research involving people living with schizophrenia, and there is a growing evidence base for CR in other mental illnesses. A case study involving the implementation and dissemination of CR within an MHS is used to demonstrate the translation of theory into service development.

# ORGANIZATIONAL FACTORS THAT FACILITATE IMPLEMENTATION OF COGNITIVE REMEDIATION

At a systems level, successful implementation of CR requires organizational change as well as clinician behavioral change. Understanding the complexity of organizational processes can assist in implementation planning (Fig. 6.1).

## Organizational Culture and Climate

The successful translation of evidence based-programs (EBP) like CR from the "bench" or research settings to routine clinical services depends in part on whether the organization facilitates innovation and whether the contextual factors existing at the time of implementation are permissive of change. There is a growing awareness of the need to account for these system factors with the development of measurement tools to capture the more stable construct of organizational culture as well as the more dynamic constructs of the organizational and implementation climate (Brownson et al., 2012).

*Organizational culture* refers to what makes organizations unique; it involves shared values, shared history, and experiences (Aarons, Horowitz, Dlugosz, & Ehrhart, 2012). It can be covert and can be taught to new staff in informal interactions. Studies have found that organizational culture is relatively impermeable to

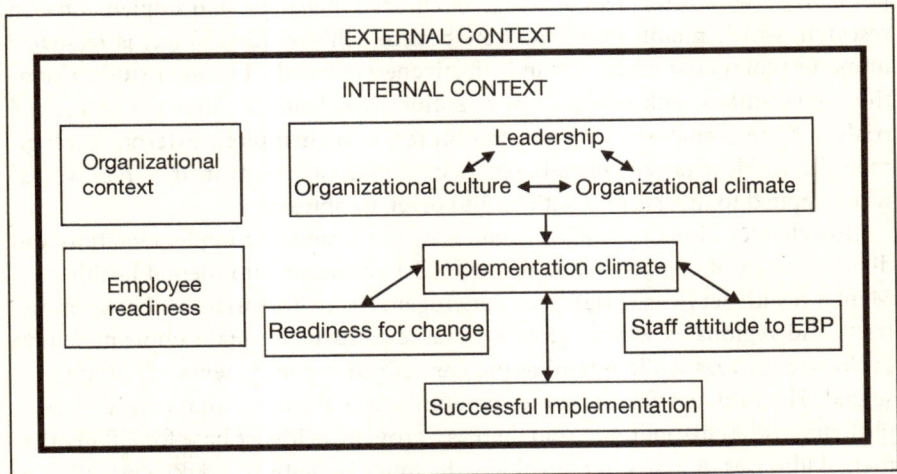

**Figure 6.1** Multiple levels of organizational processes and implementation. EBP = evidence-based practice.
Adapted from Aarons, G. S., Horowitz, J. D., Dlugosz, L. R., & Ehrhart, M. G. (2012). The role of organisational processes in dissemination research. In R. C. Brownson, Graham A. Colditz, & Enola K. Proctor (Eds.), *Dissemination and implementation research in health: Translating science into practice.* New York: Oxford University Press.

change, although organizations that are supportive of employees and able to adapt to change are more effective (Parmelli et al., 2011).

A related concept is organizational climate, which can be more fluid and potentially more malleable than organizational culture. *Organizational climate* refers to staff perceptions of management practices and the impact of these practices on their well-being (Schneider, Ehrhart, & Macey, 2011). A distinction can be made between the generic climate, defined by broad, multiple domains such as stress or autonomy, and more focused strategic climates (e.g., implementation climate) (Aarons, et al., 2012).

*Implementation climate* can be defined as "employees' shared perceptions of the importance of innovation implementation within the organisation" (Klein, Conn, & Sorra, 2001). Detailed measures of organizational climate have been developed and used in mental health settings as part of strategies to enhance the success of a program's implementation (Aarons, 2007). The implementation strategy may include leadership training for key managers, the development of policies and governance procedures, and incentives for staff with quarantined therapy time and case weighting. These strategies aimed at improving organizational climate have been found to facilitate implementation of EBP (Aarons, Horowitz, Dlugosz, & Ehrhart 2012).

## Leadership

Leadership is required to maintain and hold the CR implementation strategy over the duration of the process despite the vicissitudes of care delivery, which is affected by many variables (e.g., funding cuts). Mental health staff have been found to value the characteristics of the transformational leader (Corrigan, Steiner, McCracken, Blaser, & Barr, 2001). Transformational leaders enable staff to perform at higher levels, often by proactively encouraging professional development; acting as trusted, reliable role models; and conveying a service vision (Jung & Sosik, 2006). A brief measure of implementation leadership, the Implementation Leadership Scale (ILS), can be used as part of a multilevel implementation process (Aarons, Ehrhart, & Farahnak, 2014).

## Readiness to Change and Attitudes Toward Evidence-Based Practice

Successful implementation of CR requires change and cannot rely on individual change agents or program champions. Readiness to change needs to be considered at all levels of the organization, both individually and collectively. Organizational factors have been found to be more influential on implementation outcome than individual factors (Aarons, et al., 2012). Key change beliefs have been identified.

*Change valence* relates to the stakeholders' beliefs that the change is beneficial. In regard to CR implementation, there needs to be recognition of the role of cognition in limiting clients' functional outcome. The exponential increase in publications on the topic has raised awareness of this missing link in the therapeutic approach to psychosis (Wykes, Huddy, Cellard, McGurk, & Czobor, 2011).

In addition, clinicians are frequently confronted with the functional consequences of the cognitive impairment associated with mental illness, effects on adherence to treatment plans and community functioning.

Program champions and close alignment with academics and researchers who study cognition in psychological disorders can assist in permeating the need to address cognitive deficits throughout the organization.

*Change efficacy* refers to the degree to which employees feel capable of implementing the change. Enabling and giving staff the latitude to explore innovative, evidenced-based therapies such as CR is influenced by the organizational culture and leadership. CR champions need to outline an implementation plan that can be endorsed by the organizational executive. An implementation team can negotiate the operationalization of the plan and increase efficiency and utility of the therapy by allowing the therapist to focus on delivering the program while the implementation team is responsible for evaluation and feedback to the organization.

*Discrepancy* is the identified need for change due to a perceived gap between current service provision and the desired service. Service audits can help raise awareness of the discrepancy between recommended and actual service provision (Macpherson, Hovey, Ranganath, Uppal, & Thompson, 2008). In addition, initiatives aimed at benchmarking the use of psychosocial interventions can highlight service provision discrepancies, bringing together multiple similar services within a region to gauge comparative performance and facilitate shared learning.

An Australian clinician-led study, initiated by the perception of staff that cognitive difficulties were affecting adherence to therapy, showed a strong positive correlation between cognitive deficits, as measured by the Large Allen Cognitive Level Screen, and the medication adherence rating scale. Despite the issue noted by staff, no participant reported the use of medication adherence aids. The study team developed a CR program that linked with the participants' individual care plans, allowing for provision of medication adherence aids as needed (Cairns et al., 2013).

*Principal support* refers to the belief that those in authority and opinion leaders are consistently committed to implementation. In relation to CR, this requires particular endorsement of the program, even in settings of limited resources in which services need to choose a small number of key EBPs.

## IMPLEMENTATION DRIVERS

The successful implementation of CR within an organization requires attention to the so-called implementation drivers of leadership, support for organizational processes, and a focus on mechanisms to enhance staff competency in CR (Fig. 6.2).

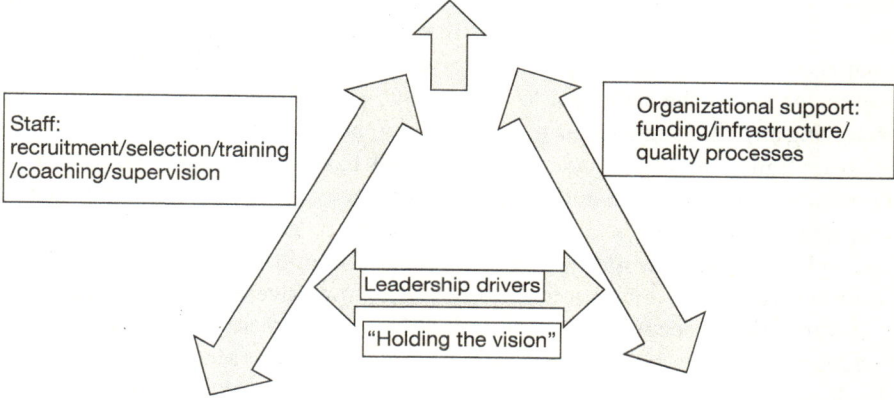

Goal: Improved functional outcomes for people diagnosed with mental illness

Initiative: Routine access to cognitive remediation therapies

Method: Strategic plan focusing on key implementation drivers

Staff: recruitment/selection/training/coaching/supervision

Organizational support: funding/infrastructure/quality processes

Leadership drivers

"Holding the vision"

**Figure 6.2** Drivers for implementation of cognitive remediation.
Adapted from Fixsen, D., Naoom, S., Blasé, K., Friedman, R., & Wallace, F. (2008). *Implementation research: A synthesis of the literature.* Tampa, FL: University of South Florida, Louis de la Parte Florida Mental Health Institute, national Implementation Research Network.

## Leadership

Executive endorsement for implementation of CR is a fundamental step in developing organizational readiness to incorporate this EBP, but leadership needs to be considered broadly.

- Senior executive management is responsible for policies and the overall organizational strategic direction. Leaders at this level should understand the need for implementing CR and, in a resource-limited environment, why this EBP needs to have priority over other innovations. Executives need to be convinced not only clinically but also on the cost benefit to the organization.
- Innovation champions need to develop a business case covering the costs in relation to recurrent staff, training, and infrastructure costs as well as anticipated benefits and cost offsets (Reeder et al., 2014).
- At the team level, team leaders and clinical directors need to be convinced to prioritize CR and allow motivated staff time for training, supervision, and delivery of CR. This may result in reallocation of cases

and a requirement for other case managers to understand and believe in the benefit of the therapy to their consumers.

Regular feedback mechanisms that reflect and are tailored to the priorities of each service level assist with embedding the process. CR participants' progress reports can be a standing agenda item at weekly clinical team meetings. This helps integrate the program into routine care, allows the team to take ownership of the program, and facilitates referrals to the program and an understanding of the resources (staff and funding) that are required to run CR. CR implementation managers need to regularly maintain a workforce map, tracking the skills and competencies of the staff pool to deliver high-quality CR and anticipating and resolving any challenges to the maintenance of the program.

Team leaders should provide regular feedback to senior managers, emphasizing the utility of the program and the impact on service outcomes, such as patients' improved independence and diminished reliance on professional care. An example of a feedback mechanism is the quarterly utilization assessment of the Neuropsychological Educational Approach to Cognitive Remediation (NEAR) program. This assessment provides executive and team leaders with objective feedback about the how the program is serving patients (Medalia, Revheim, & Herlands, 2009).

A coalition of interest groups can also assist in providing regional leadership. In Brisbane, Australia, the Brisbane Cognitive Remediation Interest Group (BCRIG) formed in 2008 at the time of training provided by Professor Alice Medalia and, on her advice, has continued to meet monthly ever since. The group provides collegiate support, advice, shared resources and training, and strategic organizational advice.

## Organizational Processes

Innovative change practices need facilitative organizational processes. Most health-related services are required to measure activity and risk. Clinical governance processes can involve regular audits that track and report on core components of treatments as recommended in therapeutic guidelines. Current MHS service contexts are characterized by an emphasis on efficiency and cost containment with high levels of accountability. Information technology, strategically used and made available, can support staff to deliver care as well as record activity in a time-efficient manner. Computer-based CR has leveraged modern technology. Organizationally, this does necessitate an investment in computers and Internet access to programs. Successful implementation, including an initial investment to embed programs, needs to be included in the budget. Given these infrastructure costs, decisions need to be made about the costs and benefits of centralizing the program or decentralizing it with satellite small programs close to where people live. A balance needs to be made between the issues of access, with concerns about sustainability, and the mantenance of fidelity in smaller outreach programs.

CR implementation will compete with other organizational priorities and requirements both internal and external to the organization (e.g., government health policies). Despite the promise of improved functioning and less reliance on the health care system, these more distal objectives can be relegated behind acute, crisis, "frontdoor" demands in an MHS. Organizations providing principal support for CR recognize that managing demand involves delivering comprehensive care that focuses on symptoms and functioning to enable people to transition to greater self-management and less reliance on specialist care. CR is a core intervention to enable improved community functioning (Dark, Cairns, & Harris, 2013).

## Changing Clinician Practice

### INTEREST IN EVIDENCE BASED PRACTICE AND COGNITIVE REMEDIATION

Staff attitudes toward EBP have been found to be a common barrier to implementation. There are multiple factors involved, including prior staff training in EBP, "marketing" of the particular EBP, staff-perceived competencies, and perceived organizational support for therapy-specific time. In Australia, 106 clinical staff members in an MHS were surveyed to ascertain their attitude toward CR and, in particular, cognitive behavioral therapy for psychosis. Fifty-one people (48.1% of staff) completed the survey. There was an interest in learning more about the cognitive impairments of psychosis, with 56.5% of respondents endorsing this item. Even more staff members (78.3%) evidenced a particular interest in training in CR awareness and cognitive compensatory strategy skills, and 39% of respondents had already attended CR training. These results validated the development of tiered training modules targeting cognitive therapies.

### ABSORPTIVE CAPACITY

At an organizational level and at the staff level, there is a finite capacity to accommodate change and innovation. Formal change processes include staging and pacing innovations. Within services, there can be a perception from staff that they are required to do more with less. A business case for implementation needs to include a justification for why a CR program should be run by the service, identification of the need to be addressed, the opportunity costs or benefits to the organization, and the utility of the program within the particular service context. Incentives to staff and, at times, to organizations can increase absorptive capacity. Staff incentives can take the form of recognized therapy-specific time, support to attend CR conferences, and caseload weightings. Organizational benefits can include retention of skilled staff within a service and a reputation for innovation and quality service provision.

### TRAINING, COACHING, AND SUPERVISION

There is limited but growing research into the effectiveness of staff training in delivering EBPs. Distinctions can be made between knowledge or awareness training and skill acquisition or competency training. Research into training in psychosocial treatments has found that didactic teaching on its own is inadequate (Beidas & Kendall., 2010). Multifaceted training informed by adult learning principles requires an integrated approach wherein didactic components are complemented by skills training involving experiential learning and opportunities to practice skills. Training also needs to be tiered within an organization and should include the following components:

- Awareness training in cognitive therapies for managers who determine therapy, training time, and case weighting
- Awareness training for staff who do not want to be therapists or facilitators but who are often a referral source and are essential in integrating and sustaining gains into clients' day-to-day functioning
- Novice practitioner training that assumes a need for ongoing supervision of practice
- CR-experienced practitioner training and training for specialists in the field, which may include modules on supervision and research techniques

A therapist capability framework for CR can be developed and should articulate not only the rated skill level but also the responsibilities of the various levels of management (Table 6.1).

## Who, What, and When to Train

Training is best molded to strategic outcomes. When an MHS seeks to implement CR, training of MHS staff should target understanding of cognition in mental illness, treatment approaches, referral pathways, and how to reinforce and integrate CR into the overall recovery and treatment plan. To some extent, this type of training can be provided efficiently with the use of modern technology, such as Web-based computer platforms (Cairns, 2014). Awareness training targeted at middle and senior managers should focus on an understanding of how improved functional outcomes linked to CR may assist in overall service aims (e.g., mainstreaming stabilized patients) and how investment in staff training and therapy time helps enable these outcomes.

Training of therapists and program facilitators requires a greater investment of time and money. Moreover, these costs may need to be recurrent as staff turnover necessitates ongoing training to maintain a critical mass of therapists to maintain a program. In 2008, twenty-six Australian mental health workers received intensive CR training over 4 days from Professor Alice Medalia. After 4 years, only two of the originally trained staff continued to deliver CR. In this situation, I have continued to train new facilitators to maintain the programs. Access to accredited training may make ongoing training expensive and may present a barrier to sustaining programs over time. CR training curriculums have been developed for

Table 6.1. COGNITIVE REMEDIATION (CR) STAFF CAPABILITY DOCUMENT

| Capability Component | Fundamental Clinician | CR Novice Practitioner | CR-Experienced Clinician | Specialist CR Therapist |
|---|---|---|---|---|
| Knowledge and skills | Aware of cognitive deficits of psychosis. Able to advise on compensatory strategies | Able to deliver CR under supervision | Proficient in delivering CR as sole practitioner or as supervisor of novice practitioner | Intensively trained with ongoing maintenance of practice and abreast of evidence base for CR |
| Supervision and credentials | Core practice supervision | Supervised practice until proficient | Participates in peer supervision and maintenance of CR practice | Endorsed to train staff in CR Able to monitor program fidelity |
| CR practice role | Able to explain CR and make appropriate referrals | Co-facilitates groups and attends supervision regularly | Facilitator, supervisor | Leadership role concerning CR in the organization Advocates for maintenance of programs and instigates research concerning CR |
| CR education role | Completes the psychosocial aspects of psychosis training (PSI) & e-learning module on cognition and psychosis | Incorporates cognitive factors in case formulation and treatment planning Collects evaluation data | Assesses new referrals. Able to coach and supervise novice practitioners | Involved in training facilitators, coaching, and supervision Supervises the experienced clinicians |
| Manager support | Support attendance at training | Supports attendance at training and supervision | Therapy and supervision time quarantined | Allocated time to manage the program, including therapy, coaching, and supervision time |
| Research and EBP role | | Keeps abreast of literature on CR | Involved in evaluation of programs and maintenance of program fidelity | Facilitates CR research and evaluation |

CR = cognitive remediation; EBP = evidence-based practice; PSI = Psychosocial Interventions.

NEAR and in the United Kingdom (Medalia et al., 2009; Reeder & Wykes, 2011). These training programs include competency assessment, but criteria to maintain credentialing over time are yet to be defined. In Australia, yearly 1-day seminars have been instigated for experienced facilitators to assist them in maintaining skills and incorporating developments in the field into practice. These seminars combine didactic presentations with peer-based supervision.

The content of training for novice practitioners should include familiarization with the particular CR program being implemented and understanding of the cognitive deficits of mental illness, mental health rehabilitation, education and adult learning theory, and motivation theory (Medalia et al., 2009) (Box 6.1).

Trainees ideally should begin practice as soon as possible after training to reinforce learning and avoid decay of skills and knowledge. In addition, practice

---

Box 6.1

BRISBANE COGNITIVE REMEDIATION INTEREST GROUP
CURRICULUM—COURSE OUTLINE

The 2-day introduction training and observed practice are prerequisites to being credentialed as a cognitive remediation (CR) facilitator. Credentialed facilitators receive ongoing monthly group supervision.

Day 1

- Introduction to CR
- Definition of cognition, neurocognition, social cognition
- Cognition and psychosis
- Cognition and function
- Therapies aimed at improving function in people living with psychosis
- The brain and psychosis
- Theoretical models for CR
- CR approaches
- Therapist qualities

Day 2

- Intake and assessment
- Treatment planning
- Bridging
- Fidelity, supervision
- Common problems
- Program evaluation

---

coaching and supervision should be provided until proficiency is reached, as assessed subjectively and by observation of practice by a specialist in the field.

The potential role of peers as co-facilitators of CR programs has not been evaluated. One site in Brisbane has routinely involved peer workers to assist engagement of new participants and to instill hope by sharing their experiences of being involved in the program. Support and supervision are given to these consumers. There is also a role for consumer-led research in CR (Rose et al., 2008).

## STAGES OF COGNITIVE REMEDIATION IMPLEMENTATION

Five stages of implementation have been described, with different priorities and challenges at each stage. These are displayed in Figure 6.3. The timeline for implementation is 2 to 4 years.

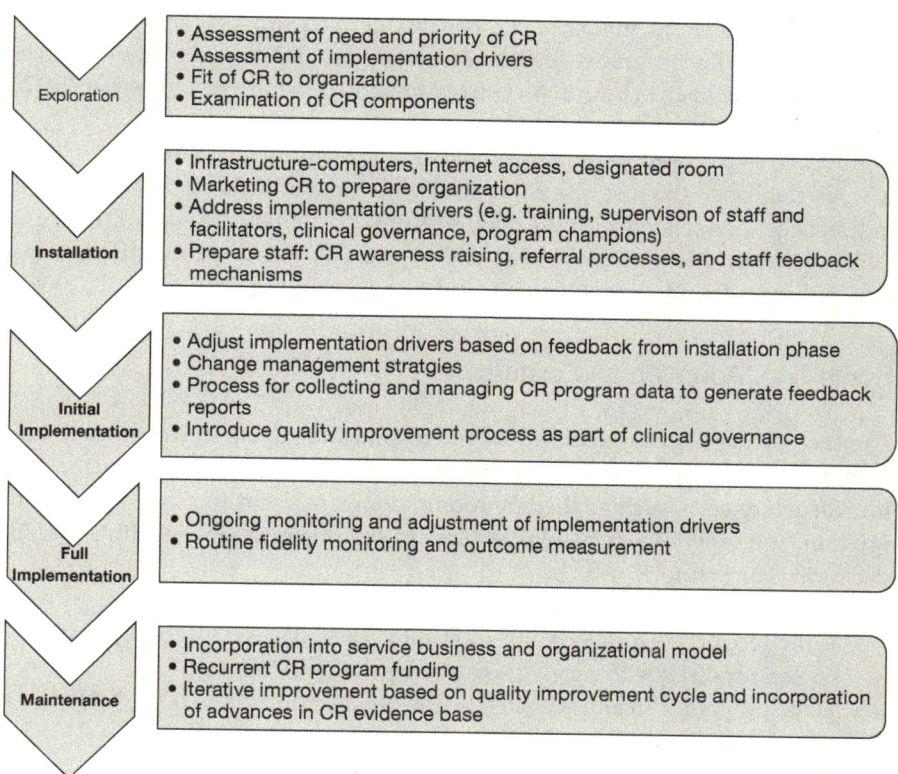

**Figure 6.3** Stages in implementation of a cognitive remediation program over a period of 2 to 4 years.

## Stage One: Exploration

The priorities in the first stage are to assess the need for CR. The imperative to implement strategies to address the cognitive deficits of schizophrenia has been well articulated:

- Cognitive impairments are the core feature of the illness; they are lifelong and are the best predictors of disability.
- Current pharmacotherapy for psychosis is not effective in addressing the cognitive deficits (Keefe et al., 2007).
- CR has evidence of effectiveness from multiple meta-analyses of randomized controlled trials (Wykes et al., 2011).
- The suboptimal outcomes of current treatments for clinical symptoms of schizophrenia have not been able to significantly alter the costs to clients, their families, society, and the economy (Sevy & Davidson, 1995).

Advocacy is required from opinion leaders and CR champions. In addition to the arguments listed earlier, improvements in basic cognition (e.g., attention, memory) are likely to influence the benefits derived from higher-order interventions, including cognitive behavioral therapies, and to improve adherence to treatment regimens (Bowie, McGurk, Mausbach, Petterson, & Harvey, 2012; Penadés et al., 2012).

Advocates also need to make a financial argument for the benefits of CR. It is well established that cognitive impairment is a major factor in the direct and indirect costs associated with the diagnosis of schizophrenia (Sevy & Davidson, 1995). A study examining the cost-effectiveness of CR in people living with schizophrenia found better outcomes and no additional costs (Patel et al., 2006).

## Stage Two: Adoption and Installation

The second stage is characterized by the organizational, structural, and instrumental changes required to implement CR. The CR business plan needs to include infrastructure costs such as therapy rooms, computers and Internet access, and program sourcing. The particular features of the organization are influential in decisions. For example,

- Is the program centralized and accessed via affordable transport systems or decentralized with access close to the person's community?
- Is the program run and operated by the organization, or does the MHS enter into a partnership with the nongovernmental organization to provide training and supervision of their staff?

An implementation team can help with multilevel engagement, monitoring fidelity, and program outcomes, aligning systems by using referral pathways and anticipating and resolving barriers to implementation.

## Stage Three: Initial Implementation

The challenges in the third stage can include program inertia with decay in the initial enthusiasm and resistance to change. The initial marketing of the programs may have set up administrators to have unrealistic expectations of the fledging programs, particularly if the expected time frame of innovation was not well explained and inadequate attention was given to communicating with members of the organizational executive. Proactive initiatives at this stage include implementation of systems to manage data and to enable efficient reporting of program outcomes and service utilization (Medalia et al., 2009). Regular program audits can become part of routine improvement cycles embedding fidelity checks and quality assurance activities.

## Stage Four: Full Implementation

In the fourth stage, the program is accepted as part of expected care. Quality assurance mechanisms have become part of regular clinical governance procedures. The challenge is to continue to adapt the programs to incorporate emerging research evidence and to respond to external factors such as funding and altered organizational priorities.

## Stage Five: Maintaining and Sustaining the Program

The final stage of implementation is achieved when the program is incorporated into the service core business. In practice, this involves mechanisms for ongoing funding and maintenance of quality improvement processes. Programs remain invigorated by sharing successes and developing partnerships, such as with vocational agencies. The challenges continue, with issues including skill retention secondary to staff turnover and external influences on organizational direction and leadership over which there may be limited influence.

## BARRIERS TO IMPLEMENTATION AND SUGGESTED SOLUTIONS

### Organizational Barriers

There needs to be an organizational strategy that is informed by marketing techniques to get stakeholders to "buy into" the new program. Many factors need to be analyzed, both external to the organization and internally, to look for possible points of leverage. Where motivations can be triangulated or converge, there is often a greater chance of success. For example, cognitive impairment has been associated with the need for extended tertiary mental health care (Reeder, Harris, Picjles, Patel, Cella, & Wykes, 2014). This has implications organizationally in terms of managing demand for services and costs. For the clinician, cognitive impairment has also been associated with poor adherence to treatment plans. Untreated cognitive impairment can result in inability to attain optimal autonomy and community functioning. Even times of organizational crisis can be opportunities for the service to review how care is delivered and to be more open to innovation, especially where there is the potential to improve efficiency, effectiveness, and costs. Economic evaluations of CR can assist in promoting systematic implementation of CR (Reeder et al., 2014).

## Staff Competency, Retention, Supervision, and Interdisciplinary Conflict

CR facilitators can come from any mental health discipline as long as they are prepared to train and have their practice supervised. Staff turnover and facilitator retention can become a major threat to sustaining the programs. A recurrent training schedule to ensure an optimal number of facilitators is recommended but can be difficult or expensive to provide. Development of online training for CR facilitators will help further dissemination and maintenance of these programs. One recently developed Web site (www.TeachRecovery.com) provides some aspects of CR training.

Ideally, supervision should occur weekly until competence is reached, then fortnightly or monthly. The structure of supervision depends on the program, the specifics of the group, and the experience of the facilitators (Medalia et al., 2009). Supervisor training was part of a Japanese CR dissemination study (Ikezawa et al., 2011).

## Inadequate Allocation of Clinician Time for Conducting Cognitive Remediation

As a general guideline, therapists need to allocate 45 minutes to facilitate the session and a further 30 minutes in preparation time. At each site, there needs to be a site program manager who is responsible for the technology and for referrals and collation of program evaluations. The program manager needs additional time, which will vary depending on the number of programs running at the site.

It is possible for different facilitators to facilitate on different days. This does require a communication strategy or protocol, but it has the advantage of enabling managers to schedule staff who may have other clinical duties. Involvement of many staff members may assist in the acceptance of CR by the team (Medalia et al., 2009).

## Inadequate Funding

The implementation literature acknowledges the importance of funding programs for successful implementation (Fixsen et al., 2005). The implementation plan and evaluation need to include funding proposals with calculation of a recurrent budget to maintain and develop the programs.

## Failure to Adapt: Context, New Evidence, and Evaluation

It is likely that ongoing CR effectiveness research and cognitive neuroscience research will produce evidence that has implications for the delivery of CR in MHSs. Regular peer supervision for experienced CR facilitators, involvement in CR research, and attendance at key CR conferences can be part of a CR therapist's performance plan and provide a process by which professional standards in CR are maintained and enhanced, enabling key staff to stay abreast of new evidence. In a CR capability framework (see Table 6.1), it is the role of the CR specialist to oversee iterative program improvements.

## CASE STUDY: IMPLEMENTATION AND DISSEMINATION OF COGNITIVE REMEDIATION WITHIN A MENTAL HEALTH SERVICE IN AUSTRALIA

In 2013, an MHS in an Australian metropolitan city with a catchment population of approximately 950,000 people structurally reorganized to facilitate EBP. Because of training by Professor Alice Medalia in 2008, the service already had CR available but only in one of the three geographic districts and with limited reach, distribution, and access. The organizational restructuring represented senior management endorsement to upscale these programs. At that time, I commenced a PhD project examining the implementation and dissemination of cognitive therapies for psychosis within the service.

In the exploration phase, endorsement was obtained from the service executive and clinical managers for service-wide implementation of CR. Staff members were surveyed before the service reorganization to ascertain their baseline knowledge and attitudes toward CR. The survey identified an existing awareness and interest in CR and a need to focus on training and supervision and on infrastructure support to acquire computers and Internet access.

In the installation stage, an implementation team was formed that met formally once a month and reported to the service Therapies Oversight Committee and Clinical Council. Tiered training was provided on the psychosocial aspect of psychosis to all staff, commencing with the team leaders, who then enlisted all clinicians to attend this fundamental training. An online e-learning module was developed to provide an introduction to cognitive aspects of psychosis for all staff members (Cairns, 2014). CR facilitator skills training workshops were held every 6 months. Potential facilitators were credentialed after attending this training and having their observed practice endorsed by an experienced CR facilitator. All programs were evaluated with the use of quarterly utility data and clinical outcome measures. One year after the service restructure and enactment of the

CR implementation plan, each geographic district had at least one CR program running, and the service had fifty-one trained facilitators.

In the initial implementation stage, adjustments were made in the supervision structure based on facilitator feedback, which indicated that centralized, service-wide supervision did not adequately meet the needs of local sites. The program was changed to provide monthly supervision to each site and a yearly service-wide CR forum to enable shared learning.

As the CR program moved into the full implementation stage, the priorities were to secure recurrent program funding and to ensure fidelity and maintenance of program quality. Routine program audits and fidelity checks were undertaken every 6 months.

Future goals for the maintenance phase were formulated, including development of CR specialists who could be trained as CR trainers and who could continue to evaluate and adapt the programs based on local outcomes and incorporating the developing CR evidence base.

## COGNITIVE REMEDIATION IN CULTURALLY AND ETHNICALLY DIVERSE POPULATIONS

Many countries, such as Britain, the United States, and Australia, are multicultural. Examples of adapting CR to a minority cultural group have been published (Press, 2011). In addition, CR has been adopted in a number of countries in Europe, Asia, and the Middle East. The goal of CR is to improve community functioning, and it follows that the needed adaptations to the program will depend on the community and cultural context. There have been two main approaches to cultural adaptation of CR: (a) creating new programs and building an associated evidence base or (b) translating existing EBP programs into the cultural context.

There are structured methods of modifying EBP to meet the needs of cultural groups (Cabassa, Baumann, & Ana, 2013). Adaptations can be made at the surface level, such as translating the language of the intervention and changing the ethnicity or appearance of role models. More sophisticated adaptations address the values, beliefs, and norms of the ethnic group and modify the intervention to take into account these cultural norms and values. The essential caveat is fidelity to the core components of the program, which are the essence of the evidence base. Any modifications need to be documented and included in the evaluation of the intervention.

The cultural adaptation process involves the following steps:

1. Translation of the protocol to align with the language and culture, as well as back-translation, with a panel of experts to examine equivalence criteria
2. Examination of the conceptual framework, with an expert panel to review the protocol session changes
3. Focus groups, with in-depth analysis by experts and participants

There are examples in which CR computer-based exercises have undergone language translation, with local facilitators embedded in the local culture delivering the cultural adaptations. Software providers have included Marker Software (COGPACK), Scientific Brain Training Pro, and PositScience.

An alternative approach is to develop a new program within the culture or ethnic group and then build an evidence base around that program. The main barriers in this approach are the higher cost and the time needed to build the evidence base (Cabassa et al., 2013).

## IMPLEMENTING THERAPIES TO ADDRESS SOCIAL COGNITION

Many of the principles and theories discussed in this chapter can be applied to other therapies. The evidence base for social cognition is still emerging, and there has been only one meta-analysis of nineteen controlled trials involving 692 participants (Kurtz & Richardson, 2012). Concerns about the limited evidence base need to be balanced against the poor social outcomes for many people with psychosis and consumer concerns about their social functioning. In an Australian national survey of people living with psychotic illness the three highest future concerns were the social outcomes of finances, social relationships, and work (Morgan et al., 2012). It can be anticipated that cultural adaptations will be more problematic for social cognition interventions, with challenges in transporting programs to other cultures.

Superficial translations of one social cognition program developed in the United States, known as Social Cognition and Interaction Training (SCIT), resulted in use of this program in at least two cities in Australia (Bartholomeusz & Allott, 2012; Parker, Foley, Walker, & Dark, 2013). The shared English language and the cultural "colonization" of Australia via American cultural media (e.g., television, film) facilitated this adoption. This is unlikely to be the case in other cultural and language groups. One study has addressed the cultural adaptation of a social cognition intervention (Social Cognitive Skills Training, or SCST) into Arabic (Gohar, Hamdi, El Ray, Horan, & Green, 2013). The training sessions were initially translated into Arabic by one of the authors, who received in-person supervision from one of the program developers. The availability of culturally appropriate assessment tools is also important. The primary outcome measure in the Gohar et al. study was the Arabic version of the Mayer-Salovey-Caruso Emotional Intelligence Test.

A corollary of the emerging evidence base for remediation of social cognitive deficits is that arguably less is known about the core components of social cognition therapies compared with the core components of CR. Although the domains of social cognition are reasonably well articulated, the evidence for remediation of the separate domains of social cognition varies; the best evidence is for remediation of facial affect recognition (Kurtz & Richardson, 2012; Savla, Vella, Armstrong, Penn, & Twamley, 2012). In addition, evidence on how best to construct a social cognition intervention program to address all the domains is still developing. The SCIT approach is based on three scaffolding phases, with affect processing targeted first, then social emotional processing, and finally integration of skills learned in previous phases into the client's real-life experiences (Penn et al., 2005). SCIT is delivered in a group setting. The optimal model of delivery has not been well researched, but there is less reliance on computer-delivered therapy compared with CR. SCIT uses video clips to train clients in social processing. Facial affect training has been successfully delivered to clients individually using a computer.

Given the limits of efficacy and effectiveness research for social cognition therapies, any implementation plan must focus on evaluation and the capacity of the service to adapt to new evidence as it arises. Choice of program will be influenced not just by the literature but also by which program has the best fit with the organization, including staff preferences and need for equipment such as computers. Most programs (e.g., cognitive enhancement therapy, SCIT) comprise between fifteen and forth-five sessions delivered weekly (Hogarty et al., 2004; Penn, et al., 2005).

Many aspects of the delivery of social cognition therapy are derived from cognitive behavioral strategies and focus on social processing and appraisal. There are comprehensive programs, such as cognitive enhancement therapy, that integrate social cognition therapy with CR and psychosocial rehabilitation. Integrated programs are attractive as service models, but it can be difficult to disentangle the core effective components.

## CONCLUSIONS

There is a consensus among consumers, caretakers, clinicians, researchers, policymakers, and government representatives that outcomes from severely disabling mental illnesses such as schizophrenia are suboptimal. The domains of impairment in schizophrenia (i.e., positive symptoms, negative symptoms, neurocognition, and social cognition) have been well articulated. Research continues to deliver evidence-based treatments that fail to be available in routine mental health care. Further discovery research is required to develop and refine effective treatments for schizophrenia, but attention also needs to be focused on developing systems that can rapidly incorporate current and ongoing research into practice. The emerging field of implementation science can inform this translation of evidence "from bench to bedside." Clinicians and service managers need to have skills in the critical appraisal of effectiveness research but also skills in effective implementation of evidence.

Improving the functional outcomes for people diagnosed with schizophrenia requires routine access to therapies addressing cognitive impairment. CR is an evidence-based treatment that should be routinely available. Realizing this goal requires an organizational systems approach that is informed by implementation science.

# REFERENCES

Aarons, G. A. (2007). Transformational and transactional leadership: Association with attitudes toward evidence-based practice. *Psychiatric Services, 57*(8), 1162–1169.

Aarons, G. A., Ehrhart, M. G., & Farahnak, L. R. (2014). The Implementation Leadership Scale (ILS): Development of a brief measure of unit level implementation leadership. *Implementation Science, 9*(45), 9–45.

Aarons, G. A., Horowitz, J. D., Dlugosz, L. R., & Ehrhart, M. G. (2012). The role of organizational processes in dissemination and implementation research. In Ross C. Brownson, Graham A. Colditz, & Enola K. Proctor (Eds.), *Dissemination and implementation research in health: Translating science into practice.* New York: Oxford University Press.

Bartholomeusz, C. F., & Allott, K. (2012). Neurocognitive and social cognitive approaches for improving functional outcome in early psychosis: Theoretical consideration and current state of evidence. *Schizophrenia Research and Treatment.* doi:10.1155/2012/815315

Beidas, R. S., & Kendall, P. C. (2010). Training therapists in evidence-based practice: A critical review of studies from a systems-contextual perspective. *Science and Practice, 17*, 1–30.

Bowie, C. R., McGurk, S. R., Mausbach, B., Petterson, T. L., & Harvey, P. D. (2012). Combined cognitive remediation and functional skills training for schizophrenia: Effects on cognition, functional competence, and real-world behaviour. *American Journal of Psychiatry, 169*, 710–718.

Brownson, R., Colditz, G., & Proctor, E. (2012). *Dissemination and implementation research in health: Translating science into practice.* New York: Oxford University Press.

Cabassa, L., Baumann, A., & Ana, A. (2013). A two-way street: Bridging implementation science and cultural adaptations of mental health treatments. *Implementation Science, 8*(1), 1–14.

Cairns, A. (2014). Cognition in mental health and the impact on day-to-day functioning. Retrieved from www.teachrecovery.com

Cairns, A., Hill, C., Dark., F., McPhail, S., & Marion, G. (2013). The Large Allen Cognitive Level Screen as an indicator for medication adherence among adults accessing community mental health services. *The British Journal of Occupational Therapy, 76*(3), 137–143.

Corrigan, P. W., Steiner, L., McCracken, S. G., Blaser, B., & Barr, M. (2001). Strategies for disseminating evidence-based practices to staff who treat people with serious mental illness. *Psychiatric Services, 52*(12), 1598–1606.

Dark, F., Cairns, A., & Harris, H. (2013). Cognitive remediation: The foundation of psychosocail treatment of schizophrenia. *Australian and New Zealand Journal of Psychiatry, 47*(6), 505–507.

Fixsen, D., Naoom, S., Blasé, K., Friedman, R., & Wallace, F. (2005). *Implementation research: A synthesis of the literature.* Tampa, FL: University of South Florida, Louis de la Parte Florida Mental Meath Institue, National Implementation Research Network.

Gohar, S. M., Hamdi, E., El Ray, L. A., Horan, W. P., & Green, M. F. (2013). Adapting and evaluating a social cognitve remediation program for schizophrenia in Arabic. *Schizophrenia Research, 148*(1–3), 12–17.

Hogarty, G. E., Flesher, S., Ulrich, R., Greenwald, D., Pogue-Geile, M., Kechavan, M., . . . & Zoretich, R. (2004). Cognititve enhancement therapy for schizophrenia: Effects of a 2-year randomized trial on cognition and behavior. *Archives of General Psychiatry*, *61*(9), 866–876.

Ikezawa, S., Mogami, T., Hayami, Y., Sato, I., Kato, T., Kimura, I., Pu, S., . . . & Nakagome, K. (2011). The pilot study of a neuropsychological educational approach to cognitive remediation for patients with schizophrenia in Japan. *Psychiatry Research*, *195*(3), 107–110.

Jung, D., & Sosik, J. J. (2006). Who are the spellbinders? Identifying personal attributes of charismatic leaders. *Journal of Leadership and Organisational Studies*, *12*(4), 12–26.

Keefe, R. S. E., Bilder, R. M., & Davis, S. M., Harvey, P. D., Palmer, B. D., Gold, J. M., . . . & Neurocognitive Working Group. (2007). Neurocognitive effects of antipsychotic medications in patients with chronic schizophrenia in the CATIE trial. *Archives of General Psychiatry*, *64*, 633–647.

Klein, K. J., Conn, A. B., & Sorra, J. S. (2001). Implementing computerized technology: An organisational analysis. *Journal of Applied Psychology*, *86*(6), 811–824.

Kurtz, M., & Richardson, C. L. (2012). Social cognitve training for schizophrenia: A meta-analytic investigation of controlled controlled research. *Schizophrenia Bulletin*, *38*(5), 1092–1104.

Macpherson, R., Hovey, N., Ranganath, K., Uppal, A., & Thompson, A. (2008). NICE guidelines on treating schizophrenia—Audit. *Psychiatric Bulletin*, *32*(75). doi:10.1192/pb.32.2.75

Medalia, A., Revheim, N., & Herlands, T. (2009). *Cognitive remediation for psychological disorders: Therapist guide*. Treatments That Work series. New York: Oxford University Press.

Morgan, V., Waterreus, A., Jablensky, A., Mackinnon, A., McGrath, J. J., Carr, V., . . . & Saw, S. (2012). People living with psychotic illness 2010: Report on the second national mental health survey. *The Australian and New Zealand Journal of Psychiatry*, *46*(8), 735–752.

Parker, S., Foley, S., Walker, P., & Dark, F. (2013). Improving the social cognitive deficits in schizophrenia: A community trial of Social Cognition and Interaction Training (SCIT). *Journal of Australasian Psychiatry*, *21*(4), 346.

Parmelli, E., Flodgren, G., Beyer, F., Bailie, N., Schaafsma, M. E., & Eccles, M. P. (2011). The effectiveness of strategies to change organisational culture to improve healthcare performance: A systematic review. *Implementation Science*, *6*(33), 1–8.

Patel, A., Everitt, B., Knapp, M., Reeder, C., Grant, D., Ecker, C., & Wykes, T. (2006). Schizophrenia patients with cognitive deficits: Factors associated with costs. *Schizophrenia Bulletin*, *32*(4), 776–785.

Penadés, R., Catalán, R., Pujol, N., Masana, G., García-Rizo, C., & Bernardo, M. (2012). The integration of cognitive remediation therapy into the whole psychosocial rehabilitation process: An evidence-based and person-centered approach. *Rehabilitation Research and Practice*. doi:10.1155/2012/386895

Penn, D. L., Roberts, D. L., Munt, E. D., Silerstein, E., Jones, N., & Sheitman, B. (2005). A pilot study of social cogntion and interaction training (SCIT) for schizophrenia. *Schizophrenia Research*, *80*(2–3), 357–359.

Press, C. J. (2011). *Developing culturally adapted cognitive remediation for South Asian first episode psychosis sufferers* (Unpublished doctoral dissertation). The Faculty of Medical and Human Sciences, University of Manchester, U.K.

Reeder, C., Harris, V., Picjles, A., Patel, A., Cella, M., & Wykes, T. (2014). Does change in cognitive function predict change in costs of care for people with a schizophrenia diagnosis? *Schizophrenia Bulletin, 40*(6), 1472–1481.

Reeder, C., & Wykes, T. (2011). *CIRcuITS* (version 2.1.7). Spika Ltd., London.

Rose, D., Farrier, D., Doran, A. M., Sporle, T., Bogner, D., & Wykes, T. (2008). What do clients think of cognitive remediation therapy?: A consumer-led investigation of satisfaction and side effects. *American Journal of Psychiatric Rehabilitation, 11*, 181–204.

Savla, G. N., Vella, L., Armstrong, C. C., Penn, D. L., & Twamley, E. W. (2012). Deficits in domains of social cognition in schizophrenia: A meta-analysis of the empirical evidence. *Schizophrenia Bulletin, 39*, 979–992.

Schneider, B., Ehrhart, M. G., & Macey, W. A. (2011). Achievements and the road ahead. In M. N. Ashkanasy, C. P. M. Wilderom, & M. F. Peterson (Eds.), *Handbook of organisational culture and climate* (pp. 29–49). Newbury Park, CA: Sage.

Sevy, S., & Davidson, M. (1995). The cost of cognitive impairment in schizophrenia. *Schizophrenia Research, 17*, 1–3.

Wykes, T., Huddy, V., Cellard, C., McGurk, R., & Czobor, P. (2011). A meta-analysis of cognitive remediation for schizophrenia: Methodology and effect sizes. *American Journal of Psychiatry, 168*(5), 472–485.

# 7

# Addressing Cognitive Distortions, Dysfunctional Attitudes, and Low Engagement in Cognitive Remediation

CHRISTOPHER R. BOWIE AND MAYA GUPTA ■

## INTRODUCTION

Creating our own reality by interpreting meaning in everyday events is a normal part of daily life. We are constantly evaluating our experiences in order to make sense of the world and ourselves. These thinking patterns are malleable; for example, biology and past experiences can shape the ways in which we appraise the events in our lives and our predictions about the future. In this chapter, these *patterns of thinking* are referred to as "cognitions," whereas a person's *cognitive processing abilities* are referred to as "neurocognition." Although cognitions and consequent distortions of reality are ubiquitous, distorted thinking patterns can become pervasive and debilitating for individuals who experience severe mental illness. Maladaptive thinking styles can permeate multiple domains of a person's life and frequently emerge as important treatment targets in therapy. It comes as no surprise, then, that these insidious thinking styles also emerge during cognitive remediation (CR).

We hope that this chapter will illuminate common maladaptive thinking styles and dysfunctional attitudes that may manifest during CR. In it, we share some strategies for addressing these beliefs *with the intent of promoting patient engagement in CR*, not as a guide on how to alter patients' negative attitudes or core beliefs. Some patients may require more intensive cognitive therapies, such as cognitive behavioral therapy (CBT), in tandem with CR.

## UNDERSTANDING COGNITIVE DISTORTIONS
## AND DYSFUNCTIONAL ATTITUDES

So what are cognitive distortions, exactly? This section describes cognitive distortions and dysfunctional attitudes and the roles these thoughts play in CR.

To understand cognitive distortions, it is helpful to go back to the original cognitive model proposed by Aaron Beck more than half a century ago (Beck, 1967, 1979). Beck developed cognitive therapy, which was a type of psychotherapy for depression in which depressive symptoms were conceptualized as resulting from dysfunctional thinking patterns. Cognitive therapy aimed to improve mood and behavior by addressing and modifying these underlying dysfunctional thoughts and beliefs. Since its inception, cognitive therapy has been rigorously tested and evaluated, has undergone several modifications, and is now broadly applied to a diverse range of psychological disorders. A full presentation of this model and its treatment techniques is beyond the scope of this chapter but can be found in other sources.

The cognitive model proposed by Beck involves three levels of thought: core beliefs, underlying assumptions, and automatic thoughts. *Core beliefs* are fundamental beliefs one has about oneself, other people, and the world. These beliefs are often developed at an early age and are seen as truths about the way things are. *Underlying assumptions* (or, as we will refer to them here, *dysfunctional attitudes*) are attitudes, rules, and expectations that stem from core beliefs. Underlying assumptions often take the form of "if . . . then" statements (e.g., "If I make a mistake, then I am a total failure"). *Automatic thoughts* are situation-specific thoughts that can lead to a particular emotional response or behavior. Automatic thoughts can sometimes be fleeting, innocuous thoughts such as "What will I have for dinner tonight?", but they can also be more intense, negative thoughts such as "I can't believe I messed this up again." Negative automatic thoughts are a form of cognitive distortion that can be traced back to particular underlying assumptions and maladaptive core beliefs.

It is important to note that people develop coping responses, both adaptive and maladaptive, to deal with their core beliefs, dysfunctional attitudes, and cognitive distortions. Both the thoughts and their associated behavioral coping responses (e.g., avoidance) often come to light during CR.

Some CR paradigms do not specifically address the role that cognitions play in neurocognition, but we argue that these thoughts and beliefs can act as a significant barrier to CR treatment success. This is particularly salient when one considers whether and how people transfer their neurocognitive gains to changes in everyday behavior. How can we expect translation of cognitive gains to real-world behaviors when maladaptive thought patterns continue to perpetuate feelings of doubt and undermine one's confidence?

People tend to have several types of cognitive distortions. Table 7.1 identifies common maladaptive cognitive distortions and examples of how they may manifest in CR. This table also provides examples that are intended to help the therapist reframe these cognitive distortions in a way that redirects the patient's attention to the CR activity. In sessions, it can be helpful to work with patients to help them identify their automatic thoughts by using a worksheet. Forms 7.1 and 7.2 provide an example of such a worksheet and how it might be completed by a patient with therapist guidance.

Unlike typical CBT (in which therapists and patients collaboratively identify the links between thoughts, mood, and behavior; keep detailed thought records; and test of beliefs as a primary goal), CR uses these reframing techniques with the primary goal of keeping participants engaged with CR and using their neurocognition in daily life. This reframing experience may be internalized across treatment sessions, but the intention is to keep the intervention at more of a surface level. Attempts to engage in comprehensive and in-depth therapy (e.g., core belief/schema work) are unlikely to be feasible within CR sessions unless the treatment is intensive and allows for considerable work with individual patients.

## TECHNIQUES FOR COGNITIVE REMEDIATION

CR is fertile ground for cognitive distortions. These thoughts are likely to manifest in a range of activities within session and serve to limit the degree to which neurocognitive improvements make their way into positive behavior change outside of

*Table 7.1.* COMMON COGNITIVE DISTORTIONS IN COGNITIVE REMEDIATION
AND REFRAMING STATEMENTS

| Cognitive Distortion | Examples from Cognitive Remediation | Therapist Reframing |
|---|---|---|
| Black-or-white thinking | "I am a failure because I can't do this perfectly." | "Some of these exercises are quite difficult. Remember, it's important that we challenge ourselves in order to develop new abilities and strategies." |
| Labeling | "I'm too dumb." | "Getting a low score can be upsetting, but everyone has different strengths and areas of difficulty. Finding new areas for us to train is exactly what we are hoping for." |
| Catastrophizing | "If I can't do this exercise, how can I ever return to work?" | "Remember that this is a process; you will develop your skills over time. Today's task is the next step toward reaching your goals." |
| Filtering | "I had a lucky streak, but I'm back to not being able to do it." | "It sounds like we are doing our job! We need to challenge ourselves in order to foster new learning and develop our skills." |
| Fortune telling | "I'm going to fail this one." | "That's okay. Failing is a great opportunity to reflect on our strategies and try out new ones." |

**My personal goal for today's session:**

|  |
|--|
|  |

**How today's goal relates to my overall cognitive remediation goals:**

|  |
|--|
|  |

**Here is how I took control of my thoughts to help my cognitive abilities:**

| Negative Thoughts Identified | Reframing Thoughts | Behavior Plan |
|---|---|---|
|  |  |  |
|  |  |  |
|  |  |  |
|  |  |  |

**My personal goal for today's session:**

*Improving memory skills*

*Picking up new strategies for remembering things, especially when people give me instructions by talking to me*

**How today's goal relates to my overall cognitive remediation goals:**

*Improving my memory will help me get back to work.*

**Here is how I took control of my thoughts to help my cognitive abilities:**

| Negative Thoughts Identified | Reframing Thoughts | Behavior Plan |
|---|---|---|
| This was way too hard. | I got a good workout. I guess I could try new strategies that might work. | Don't give up—keep trying this. Ask therapist or peer what strategies work for them. |
| I'm terrible at memory, so this game is going to be a disaster. | I keep saying memory is what I need to improve, so I have to keep at it. | Make sure I keep playing even if I do poorly. Take a break and catch my negative thoughts. |
| Sure, I got 80% correct here, but that would get me fired if I ever go back to work. | This is the place to make mistakes so I can get better and try new strategies—see what is not working for me right now. | Make a list of how many mistakes people make in everyday life—is it normal to make a mistake at work? |

sessions. The ability of the therapist to apply various therapeutic techniques in CR treatments is a function of his or her prior training with these techniques and the structure of the sessions (i.e., length of treatment sessions, duration of treatment, size and composition of the group). In addition to the reframing opportunities described earlier, several other methods from cognitive therapies and CBT can be applied to CR.

## Goal Setting

As with any psychotherapy, setting goals is an important part of gaining patient buy-in, monitoring progress, and making decisions about the direction of the treatment.

There are many options for how a therapist can introduce goal setting. Importantly, goal setting should be individually tailored to each person's self-identified areas for functioning. Consistent with the purpose of this book, goal setting can be an ideal way to frame CR in the context of transferring cognitive gains to higher quality of life and better everyday functional outcomes. Goals can cover several areas of functioning, but it is often helpful to provide a paper displaying the general framework that patients can refer to and take notes on, based on global domains such as self-care, household tasks, social and interpersonal functions, leisure time, vocational functioning, and community activities. To encourage participants to stay focused on their CR, it is best to start goal setting with open-ended questions and then progress to structured goal-setting exercises when necessary. It is ideal to perform goal setting in a private individual session, even if the CR sessions are being performed in a group. This might mean planning for an orientation session or setting aside time across sessions to check in with individuals. Goal setting should be a collaborative and continuous experience. That is, the therapist's role is to help patients identify their own goals, put them in their own words, and continue to revisit them throughout CR to ensure that they remain appropriate and that the CR techniques are helping the patients reach those goals.

The role of the therapist in this context is to make sure that the goals are very clearly defined, include intermediate achievements that can be used to track progress, have measurable outcomes, and are plausible given the patient's baseline abilities and highest level of achievement.

Defining goals can be a challenge for anyone. Those with mental illness might face particular struggles with identifying goals for various areas of their lives. Intrinsic factors such as social anxiety, low self-confidence, and neurocognitive impairment make it difficult to envision what might be evaluated as major life changes. Historical factors such as long gaps in productivity or social relationships can lead to atrophy of the skills needed to develop toward a larger goal. The therapist shapes the patient's goals to make sure they are clearly defined, as in the following example, in which the purpose of the therapist's comments is italicized.

PATIENT: I would like to get along with other people better.

THERAPIST: That is a great goal.

*The therapist is reinforcing and praising the self-generation of a goal.*

THERAPIST: Tell me who you would like to get along better with.

*The therapist is prompting the patient to precisely specify the target people.*

PATIENT: Mostly my two close friends. I guess my brother, but I never see him anyway.

THERAPIST: How often do you see your two friends?

*The therapist is establishing a baseline frequency.*

PATIENT: I see them about twice a week. It used to be almost every day.

THERAPIST: It sounds like a better relationship with your two close friends is a great goal, because you have a history with them and you see them regularly.

*The therapist is paraphrasing and praising the patient's movement toward a more concrete goal.*

THERAPIST: Since you don't see your brother often, what if we focused just on the two friends for now? How does that sound to you?

*The therapist is providing an open-ended statement to give the patient an opportunity to clarify and expand (rather than a closed question such as "... Does that sound fair?").*

PATIENT: OK, just those two for now.

THERAPIST: OK. Now tell me a little bit about what it means when you say better? What does it mean to get along better?

*The therapist is prompting the patient to operationally define the goal.*

PATIENT: I am hoping they don't ignore me as much when we all hang out.

THERAPIST: That is important—we've all had experiences of feeling left out.

*Here, the therapist is acknowledging the meaningfulness of the goal and normalizing it.*

THERAPIST: What would it look like to *not* ignore you?

*The therapist is allowing the patient to reframe the negative consequence of his social interactions in a way that produces a more concrete and measurable goal. The therapist here is not trying to directly reframe the goal but still is allowing the patient time to self-generate. Some patients might eventually need more direct prompting by the therapist, particularly early in goal setting.*

PATIENT: I would like them to talk to me more instead of just to each other.

THERAPIST: Great, we are moving toward a specific goal—something you want to be able to *see and hear* happen. When we link our goals to things we can see and hear, we can be more confident in tracking whether these change over time.

*The therapist is teaching the importance of operationalizing the goals in a way that is directly measurable.*

THERAPIST: What other things do people do when they are including others in their conversation?

*The therapist is moving toward intermediate goals and identifying multiple opportunities to measure change.*

**PATIENT:** I'm not sure.

**THERAPIST:** Consider us talking right now. What have I been doing while we talk?

*The therapist is assisting by removing the abstract or imaginative element and providing a concrete visual example.*

**PATIENT:** Looking at me.

**THERAPIST:** Right, so I make eye contact.

*The therapist is praising but reframing the example as a more objective behavior.*

**THERAPIST:** I also position my body toward you. Anything else?

*Here, the therapist is offering other behaviors; considering time constraints, the therapist might instead choose to continue to prompt the patient to identify the behaviors.*

**PATIENT:** Yes, you move your hands a lot.

**THERAPIST:** Yes, I do! When I make gestures like this [opens palms toward patient], what does it tell you?

*The therapist again reframes the example as a concrete behavior and asks for perspective taking.*

**PATIENT:** I guess it is my turn to speak.

**THERAPIST:** Right, so could we include that as one of the specific goals?

*By framing this conclusion as a question, the therapist is keeping the process collaborative rather than directive.*

**THERAPIST:** To see if your friends are facing you more, if they are using their gestures, or even nodding to you when you talk?

*At this point, the therapist and patient would move toward creating a written list of the behaviors and goals and then continue with a range of other goals from other domains of functioning.*

In this example, the therapist works with the patient to ensure that the patient provides multiple goals that can be measured clearly with specific behaviors. The therapist also establishes an estimate of how often the behaviors occur, such as a frequency count of the number of visits or a rating of how pleasant the interactions were.

This will lead to the next aspect of goal setting—making sure the patient and the therapist collaborate to generate small steps that are likely to be achievable in short time frames and ultimately build a set of skills to reach the larger goal. For example, it is useful to break down longer-term milestone goals such as obtaining employment into shorter-term tasks such as performing a job search, updating a resume, developing skills associated with work, receiving training, and so on. Without these intermediate goals, it can be a challenge to keep patients motivated in CR sessions that might, on the surface, seem to be less relevant to a singular final goal. It is easier for patients to find overlap with the diverse activities and themes presented across sessions if they can link them to a set of intermediate steps. This continuous linking of present and upcoming activities can be a useful way to keep participants engaged in the sessions and motivated to return.

So far, we have described goal setting in a way that might seem to be specific to functioning but is not clearly linked to what happens in CR. The therapist uses goal setting in CR to clearly capture the everyday goals, because patients often come in with a vague idea of why cognition is itself a goal. They often talk about their neurocognitive deficits in a functional manner. For example, patients who want to improve their memory often describe wanting to get better at remembering people's names. We have not yet had any patients identify increasing their percentile score on a memory test or improving their skill on a computerized CR platform as a goal! The following paragraphs present some specific methods for linking the goal-setting activities described earlier to the procedures of CR.

When used in a way that links goals to the procedures of CR, goal setting can be a critical method for engaging patients in treatment early and often. It is important to take the perspective of the patient when thinking about the value of neurocognition and the purpose of improving it. It is easy to overlook how challenging it might be for someone to link neurocognitive abilities with functional goals. It is the therapist's responsibility to guide the patient toward making these links. In goal setting, it is helpful to share patients' neurocognitive profile with them, highlighting both the strengths and the processes that are more difficult (limitations) and illustrating how both might fit with their goals. The therapist demonstrates how the activities in CR can help build on their strengths, increase their functioning in other areas, and ultimately put them in a position to move toward their goals.

An example of this active linking of neurocognitive abilities to personal goals and treatment procedures is illustrated in the case of a 42-year old man who is looking to return to work after being on psychiatric disability for 5 years. Neurocognitive testing reveals *deficits* in processing speed, working memory, and verbal memory and *strengths* in sustained attention, problem solving, and visual memory. The man is socially anxious and prefers to avoid small talk. The therapist might link the patient's goal of returning to work with his profile of deficits and strengths as follows:

> Returning to work is very important to you, and that is something we will definitely keep in mind as we do this training. If we look at where you are right now, you have some real areas of strength, like being able to stay focused, solve problems, and remember things you see or do. Those skills will help you in many types of jobs. Other areas are more difficult for you. This is not unusual. We all have some thinking skills that are better than others. What we can do in this group is try to help you capitalize on those things you already do well and train the other areas. How does that sound?

After linking the neurocognitive profile with functional goals, the therapist can link the neurocognitive deficits to the patient's expectations of what will occur in therapy. While discussing the neurocognitive domain that will be targeted, the therapist uses a direct demonstration of exercises to help the patient make a concrete connection with the purpose of CR:

> Let's take a look at this cognitive exercise on the computer. [Show task.] Do you see how this game requires us to develop speed in processing

information? That is one of the areas that was a bit lower for you, so by training on games like these, you will be able to become a bit faster with your thinking skills.

Finally, the therapist works collaboratively with the patient to link the profile of neurocognitive functions with the activities he will participate in through CR and his functional goals:

Can you think of how getting better at processing information might help you on a job? [Therapist prompts if patient does not self-generate.] Great! So, tell me in your own words how working in this training program might help you reach your long-term goal of returning to work.

## Normalizing

Have you ever noticed how hard it is to type fast without making mistakes when someone is watching you type? Or, have you ever had a harder time continuing a story once a few extra people start to pay attention to you or comment on your story? Performing skilled acts in front of others and receiving frequent feedback on one's performance produces a sense of anxiety that can distort one's perception of the performance and the progress being made—yet, this is the modal structure of a session of CR! It is thus critically important to help patients understand how the work is going to focus on strengthening their skills, rather than simply eliminating a deficit or problem. Therapists can emphasize that we all have a range of abilities and find some tasks harder than others. Patients can be dissuaded from taking a categorical view of their profile as either "impaired" or "normal" by illustrating a profile of abilities or by drawing out a continuum to contrast with such categories (Figs. 7.1 and 7.2).

When referring to cognitive distortions or dysfunctional attitudes, it might be helpful to similarly frame these along a continuum. For example, we all take shortcuts in our thinking processes. Patients' appreciation of their ability to improve these attributions (rather than change from a categorical "maladaptive" to "adaptive") can be assisted by referring to them as "risky thinking shortcuts." Therapists can provide examples of how we all use these shortcuts in our daily lives, but when they start to happen more frequently or when we apply them to a number of areas of our lives, they start to shape our behavior.

**Figure 7.1** Moving from one label to another. This model is used to illustrate the natural tendency to incorrectly dichotomize what we expect to happen in cognitive remediation.

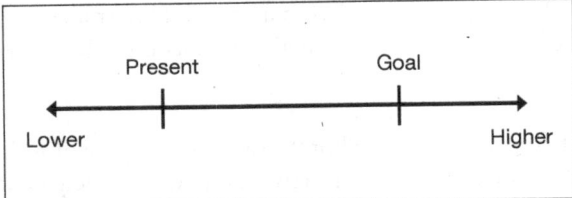

Figure 7.2 This alternative model illustrates the continuity of cognitive abilities and the goal of moving along a continuum. It can be used to provide a direct contrast to the dichotomized view to help normalize thinking about the range of abilities across domains and between people.

## Reframing "Failures" as "Challenges"

The goals of CR include challenging patients in such a way that their existing neurocognitive abilities and behavioral skills are pushed beyond their current levels of functioning. This can be an exceptionally daunting endeavor for someone with a history of low self-efficacy or perfectionistic tendencies, especially because mistakes are an inherent part of learning. One way to reframe this part of CR is to liken it to other activities in which mistakes are to be expected.

For example, consider a person who signs up for a beginner piano class. This person is expecting to be *challenged* to learn new neurocognitive and behavioral skills with a concrete goal in mind. The framing of this endeavor as a *challenge* is an adaptive way to approach what is likely to be a long series of mistakes before achieving competence. Willing engagement in the activity in order to meet a concrete goal helps keep the student motivated. Normalization procedures continue to be helpful when it comes to convincing patients in CR that not only is it normal to make mistakes but mistakes are encouraged and necessary. Framing performance around an 80% success rate as a goal helps patients appreciate the need to be challenged enough to try new ways of solving problems.

## HOW COGNITIVE DISTORTIONS MANIFEST IN COGNITIVE REMEDIATION

For people with mental illness, the gap between present and desired abilities is likely to provoke distortions and subsequent negative emotional and behavioral reactions. This might lead to minimal engagement, dropout, and lack of follow-through with using neurocognitive gains in everyday life. However, the trained therapist with basic cognitive therapy skills will anticipate, recognize, and address these distortions in order to improve the success and breadth of CR effects. In the following sections, we take the reader through three case examples of how dysfunctional attitudes might be recognized, conceptualized, and addressed in CR.

## Fictional Vignettes

These fictional case studies will help the therapist learn about some of the cognitive distortions and dysfunctional attitudes that may emerge during CR treatment. They are by no means intended to capture the full range of presenting issues but rather to give a flavor of how some of these thought patterns might manifest during treatment and how they can be effectively addressed by clinicians.

### DEPRESSION: "KAREN"

Karen is a 42-year-old woman with a longstanding history of major depressive disorder. Born into a family with four older siblings, Karen believes that she has been less successful than her older brothers and sisters. She had a few close friends in high school and has kept in touch with only one since graduating. After completing high school, Karen obtained a degree in human resources. Currently, she is experiencing a major depressive episode and has been having difficulty concentrating at work. She reports difficulties with memory, attention, and motivation. She is on leave from work but hopes to return to her previous position soon. In session, Karen sometimes expresses defeatist beliefs about her level of competence (e.g., "I can't do this") and gives up or disengages from the exercise. She often engages in self-deprecating humor to cope with difficult exercises and poor performance.

### ANXIETY: "STEVE"

Steve is a 27-year-old man who was diagnosed with obsessive compulsive disorder (OCD) at age 12. He was treated for OCD as a teenager, and although his anxiety has improved remarkably, he still has some perfectionistic tendencies. He also experiences symptoms of social anxiety and worries about what others think of him. Steve started his degree in law school but quit after his first year because of the stress. He is currently working part-time as a clerk and enjoys his job. He wants to return to law school and become a lawyer, but he believes that going back to school will only make his anxiety worse. Steve often avoids activities that he thinks might stress him out, and he is quite hard on himself when he thinks he is performing poorly. Although he has several close friends, he is apprehensive when meeting new people and is uncomfortable in groups. Steve is motivated and engaged in CR; however, in session, he speaks very little, and he keeps the difficulty level of his exercises low even when he is performing well.

### MANIA/PSYCHOSIS: "JORDAN"

Jordan is a 35-year-old man with bipolar disorder. His symptoms began to emerge in his teenage years, when he would go several nights without sleep and stay up late to work on a novel or movie script. At age 21, he moved to Los Angeles to become a movie producer. Shortly thereafter, he was hospitalized during a manic episode, and he has since returned to his hometown. Jordan reports having strained interpersonal relationships and believes that others are jealous of his talent. He is worried that his medications are affecting his concentration and creativity and preventing him from writing. He is not convinced that CR therapy will be helpful but is willing to try it. In session, Jordan continuously sets the difficulty level of his exercises too high and blames the therapist and the software program when he performs poorly.

## Case Conceptualizations and Treatment Planning

Case conceptualizations can be used to address dysfunctional attitudes and cognitive distortions that may emerge during CR treatment. They provide clinicians with a structured way in which to take into account a multitude of patient factors in order to streamline CR treatment for the patient's needs. Taking the time to develop a case conceptualization for each patient is an important tool in CR. It is helpful to complete a case conceptualization for each patient at intake and to continuously update it based on changes that occur throughout the course of treatment.

Here, we attempt to highlight some patient-specific needs for the fictional cases presented and potential ways to address these needs in session. Form 7.3 is an example of a clinician handout for case conceptualization.

### CASE CONCEPTUALIZATION FOR KAREN

*Presenting problems:*
- Depression
- Difficulty concentrating at work
- Believes that she is incompetent and less successful than others

*Patient's goals and strengths:*
- Wants to go back to work
- Successfully completed a post-secondary degree
- Has a close friend

*Cognitive distortions related to cognitive remediation:*
- "I can't do this. I'm a failure."
- "I will never get better. I will never be able to go back to work."

*Potential manifestation during cognitive remediation:*
- Gives up
- Disengages from exercise
- Drops out of treatment

*Possible solutions:*
- Provide lots of positive reinforcement.

FORM 7.3  CASE CONCEPTUALIZATION

Presenting problems:

Patient's goals and strengths:

Cognitive distortions related to cognitive remediation:

Potential manifestation during cognitive remediation:

Possible solutions:

- Normalize and encourage the challenge of experiencing "failure" on what is really just a computer exercise. This is an opportunity to learn new skills in a safe, punishment-free setting.
- Start exercises at a lower difficulty level and set parameters to increase difficulty in small steps, so that the patient can experience success in session.
- Ask the patient how she may have used some of these cognitive strategies when she was studying in school or when she was at work.

## CASE CONCEPTUALIZATION FOR STEVE

*Presenting problems:*
- Longstanding history of anxiety and perfectionistic tendencies
- Avoids activities that are perceived to be too difficult
- Socially anxious and uncomfortable in groups or around new people

*Patient's goals and strengths:*
- Wants to return to law school
- Enjoys his job
- Has positive relationships with friends

*Cognitive distortions related to cognitive remediation:*
- "Everyone here must think I am stupid. They probably make fun of me behind my back."
- "I will have a relapse if I push myself too hard."
- "I'll never get through law school."

*Potential manifestation during cognitive remediation:*
- Fails to show or cancels frequently due to anxiety
- When he does attend, keeps cognitive exercises at the easiest level
- Does not participate in group discussions

*Possible solutions:*
- Normalize and discuss the merits of making mistakes.
- Discuss therapy as a safe place to make mistakes and build skills to prepare for future career goals.
- Challenge the rationality of the thought that one mistake on a computer exercise means that he will fail out of school.
- Provide psychoeducation about how anxiety can affect cognitive performance (e.g., "inverse U"; moderate level of anxiety is good for optimal performance).
- Encourage an 80% success rate; if he gets higher than 80%, he can increase the difficulty level of the exercise.
- Provide ample positive reinforcement when he does participate in discussions.

## CASE CONCEPTUALIZATION FOR JORDAN

*Presenting problems:*

- History of manic episodes and delusions of grandiosity
- Strained interpersonal relationships; can sometimes be confrontational
- Does not buy in to the effectiveness of CR

*Patient's goals and strengths:*

- Creative, ambitious
- Motivated to improve cognition so he can continue writing

*Cognitive distortions related to cognitive remediation:*

- "This is a waste of time."
- "My therapist isn't helpful."
- "I can get better on my own, without treatment."

*Potential manifestation during cognitive remediation:*

- Sets difficulty level of exercise too high
- Blames the therapist or the computer when he performs poorly
- Dominates group discussions
- Frequently fails to show
- Disengages from the cognitive exercises
- Drops out of treatment

*Possible solutions:*

- Ask the patient to set exercise difficulty at a lower level and work his way up. If this proves difficult, see if you can pre-set the difficulty level on your software program in advance.
- Encourage the patient to consider alternative explanations for why he may have performed poorly, using gentle Socratic questioning.
- With your patients, collaboratively set group rules about participation in discussions, including not cutting others off and allowing everyone the chance to talk. If dominating of discussions continues, meet with Jordan one-on-one to discuss this and set guidelines for future sessions.
- To promote engagement in treatment, have the patient reflect on how the cognitive skills used in the computer exercises relate to his goal of writing more. Revisit his goals frequently, and tailor exercises so that he is working on relevant cognitive domains.

## SUMMARY

This chapter has presented the case for applying techniques derived from cognitive therapy and CBT in CR as a method for initiating and maintaining patient engagement and increasing the likelihood that cognitive gains will be applied in the real world despite challenges with self-confidence and motivation. Although these techniques are likely to increase the benefit of CR for many patients, they should be applied only by therapists who have received formal training in the procedures. It is important to be aware that psychological interventions are not without potential side effects (Klingberg et al., 2012) and that application of principles by weakly trained individuals can result in less effective therapy (Sholomskas et al., 2005). The methods by which therapists choose to use the principles suggested in this chapter will vary considerably, based on the setting.

If CR is conducted with a high patient-to-therapist ratio, with little time for individual attention from therapists, or on a schedule that is of short duration or includes only brief sessions, it will be more difficult to engage in the more complex techniques such as formal development and continuous setting of functional goals. Other strategies, such as catching and reframing negative self-statements, might still be feasible in this context.

We recognize that the demands of health care systems will challenge the full inclusion of cognitive therapy and CBT techniques within an existing intervention. With the increasing opportunities for patients to engage in some aspects of CR outside traditional therapeutic environments (e.g., at home using online programs), the structure of what happens *within* the CR session will continue to evolve. We argue that increasing the emphasis on the techniques described here will help move the common but incorrect perception that CR is a passive brain-training computer game and transition it to a more wholistic psychotherapy that has the chance to engage more individuals and help them translate neurocognitive improvements into positive everyday behavior change.

## REFERENCES

Beck, A. T. (1967). *The diagnosis and management of depression*. Philadelphia, PA: University of Pennsylvania Press.

Beck, A. T. (1979). *Cognitive therapy and the emotional disorders*. Penguin.

Klingberg, S., Herrlich, J., Wiedemann, G., Wölwer, W., Meisner, C., Engel, C., . . . & Wittorf, A. (2012). Adverse effects of cognitive behavioural therapy and cognitive remediation in schizophrenia: Results of the treatment of negative symptoms study. *Journal of Mental and Nervous Disease*, 200(7), 569–576.

Sholomskas, D. E., Syracuse-Siewert, G., Rounsaville, B. J., Ball, S. A., Nuro, K. F., & Carroll, K. M. (2005). We don't train in vain: A dissemination trial of three strategies of training clinicians in cognitive-behavioral therapy. *Journal of Consulting and Clinical Psychology*, 73(1), 106.

# 8

# How to Assess and Choose Computerized Cognitive Exercises

TIFFANY HERLANDS AND ALICE MEDALIA ■

## INTRODUCTION

As cognitive health becomes increasingly valued, research and clinical practice have focused on the possibility of maintaining, extending, and repairing cognitive skills. We now know that even in severe psychiatric illnesses the brain is capable of changing and developing in response to stimulation, a process known as *neuroplasticity*. Neurons adjust their activity in response to new situations or changes in the environment, and these adjustments can make cognitive processing more effective. In treatment settings, computer-based exercises are often used to provide the stimulation to facilitate neuroplasticity. Through computer-based cognitive exercises, neuroanatomical connections may be strengthened or repaired, yielding changes in neuropsychological abilities. Computers are able to provide controlled learning environments that carefully titrate the level, duration, and specific nature of cognitive stimulation. A large industry has developed to supply the demand for computer-based cognitive exercises, which are now widely available for all ages and for use in a multiplicity of settings. One setting in which they are commonly used is cognitive remediation (CR) for psychiatric patients.

Restorative CR approaches typically rely on computerized exercises that may be delivered as local, hard-drive–based software or as part of a Web-based program. These exercises are intended to provide an opportunity to practice and thereby strengthen identified areas of cognitive weakness. In any given restorative CR session, a portion of time is spent doing exercises that are intended to stimulate specific cognitive processes. The client sits in front of a computer and works on tasks that have been identified as beneficial specifically for that individual. The goal is that the client will improve not only on the exercises themselves but on the cognitive skills required to do the exercise and, most importantly, on the ability to use these skills in everyday life. For example, the goal in working on a computer task that requires memorization of words is to increase verbal memory capacity so that in everyday settings it will be easier to recall verbal information.

Clinicians offering CR must make critical decisions regarding exercise selection. With the ever-increasing availability of computer-based exercises, it has become essential for clinicians to have a theoretical and practical framework from which evaluate the usefulness and suitability of exercises for their clients and for the treatment setting in general. Because computer-based exercises are constantly being developed and improved, evaluation of available products by clinicians is a continuous process. If a CR service is to stay current and take advantage of the latest developments in technology, the clinician needs to devote time on a regular basis to consider whether newly available exercises and programs should be purchased. This chapter provides practical guidelines for making those choices and explains the theoretical framework that informs the guidelines.*

## EVALUATING A COMPUTER-BASED COGNITIVE EXERCISE

Evidence gathered across clinical and experimental research studies calls attention to three facets of a computer activity that have the potential to maximize therapeutic outcome: Does the computer activity improve the specific cognitive deficits of the patient while addressing the learning needs of the patient? Does the activity enhance generalization of cognitive skill use to functional applications? and Does the activity enhance motivation of the patient to continue to work on improving his or her cognitive health?

### What Cognitive and Learning Needs Are Addressed?

Most computer-based cognitive exercises strive to isolate and practice one cognitive skill. They are advertised as exercises to improve problem solving, executive functioning, processing speed, working memory, verbal memory, and so forth. In real life, cognitive skills are used synthetically; for example, when grocery shopping, we use verbal memory to recall the needed items, planning and organization to shop for all produce at the same time, and working memory to hold the relative merits of different products in mind while making a selection. In contrast, CR computer-based exercises typically isolate and train the component skills that we use in an integrated manner in everyday life. They do this because different people have different areas of weakness and may want to selectively strengthen particular

---

* The companies and products mentioned in this chapter are representative and are not intended to indicate a comprehensive list of products available. In referencing a product, the authors are simply using it to illustrate a feature and are not making a recommendation. The following companies and products are discussed: CIRCuiTS, Cogmed, Edmark Corporation (Thinking Things collection), Fit Brains, Lumosity, Posit Science (BrainHQ, Brain Fitness), SBTP Scientific Brain Training Pro (aka HAPPYneuron), and Sunburst Communications (Factory Deluxe).

skills (e.g., working memory). Segregating skills makes it easier to focus on training specific skills.

When evaluating computer-based cognitive training activities, it is important to do an independent assessment of the cognitive skills required by any given exercise. The manufacturer may say that the exercise targets organization, but if there is a timer that can be activated or if time figures into the score calculation, then processing speed is (or can be) also trained. Often a task requires multiple overlapping skills, or a task may be listed as targeting one skill but investigation raises questions about that categorization. The clinician needs to be familiar with the various cognitive skills and should practice the exercise while carefully thinking about what cognitive skills are being used. Sometimes it is helpful to get expert consensus—that is, to check with people trained in neuropsychology to determine whether there is consensus about what is targeted by the exercise.

## Does the Exercise Promote Generalization?

The transfer of cognitive gains to everyday life entails a process called *generalization*. The cognitive skills that are activated during CR activities start to be better utilized in other contexts, such as school, work, and home. When there is generalization of CR gains, the improvements in attention, memory, problem solving, and processing speed that are apparent on the computer programs become apparent also in real life.

A number of factors can affect generalization. Lack of opportunity to practice new cognitive skills in everyday life is an issue when patients are not actively engaged in the community (e.g., socializing, shopping, working, volunteering, attending classes). Performance anxiety, self-competency beliefs, intrinsic motivation, and an autonomy-supportive environment have been identified as other factors that affect transfer of cognitive skills (Medalia & Saperstein, 2013). Generalization may be enhanced when CR incorporates strategies to help individuals overcome barriers to transfer. These strategies can be incorporated within the computer exercises themselves, within the array of chosen exercises (see Chapter 3 on treatment planning), or within the comprehensive approach, which may include bridging discussions (see Chapter 4) and even supervised real-world experiences. We focus here on the ways in which the exercises themselves promote generalization.

According to behavioral learning theory, when a cognitive skill is exercised in a particular context, over time cues that remind the person of the context will trigger use of the cognitive skill (Shepard, 1987). For example, if a person learns to pay attention to stops on trains, he or she will also pay attention on subways and other moving vehicles. The activation of a cognitive skill is facilitated when computer tasks are contextualized in real-life situations (Cordova & Lepper, 1996). An attention task that is contextualized as responding to a target in a street scene will better promote generalization than an attention task that has no context and simply requires the individual to press a button every time a circle turns red (Choi

& Medalia, 2010). When evaluating exercises, the clinician can consider whether the skill is practiced in a context that evokes a real-life scenario. For example, is a memory task simply a list-learning task, or does it simulate a restaurant and the memory challenge to remember orders? Does the task also offer a variety of contexts (e.g., a supermarket, a social gathering, a kitchen) in addition to a restaurant? Practice of the same skill on an array of tasks that have subtly different contexts facilitates transfer of training to a wider array of novel tasks and contexts (Shepard, 1987). Therefore, clinicians can facilitate a positive treatment response by developing session plans that include a variety of tasks that challenge a specific cognitive skill in a range of increasingly complex contexts.

Providing people with strategies to maximize cognitive performance is another important way to promote generalization. An example of strategy coaching is advising someone to chunk information to enhance recall—for example, to remember all the dairy products and then all the non-foods when grocery shopping. Within a drill-and-practice computer-based exercise, there is an opportunity to apply strategies, and this can enhance task performance. At present, strategy coaching is typically delivered by therapists, who watch the patient doing an exercise and discuss the strategy. However, there have been tremendous innovations in the capacity of computers to deliver strategy coaching (Graesser, Jeon, & Dufty, 2008), and they are beginning to be applied to psychiatric populations. Some Web-based activities (e.g., CIRCuiTS; see Chapter 5) now provide strategy coaching in the form of messages to the patient. Research is needed to disentangle whether it is the therapist's delivery of strategy coaching or the strategy tips per se that work synergistically with drill-and-practice and functional skills training to enhance functional outcome.

## Is the Exercise Motivating?

Inasmuch as CR is a training activity, it relies on principles of learning, which include the role of motivation in the learning process. Self-determination theory, a widely accepted theory of motivation, articulates a broad framework guiding an understanding of the individual differences and contexts that facilitate or undermine motivated behavior (Ryan & Deci, 2000). This theory distinguishes between intrinsic and extrinsic motivation. Whereas intrinsically motivated behavior stems largely from one's enjoyment and interest in a task, extrinsically motivated behavior is driven by pursuit of outcomes separate from the task, such as rewards or punishments linked to the behavior or the task. A computer exercise that is designed to be fun and interesting promotes intrinsic motivation; an exercise that is designed with points and rewards promotes extrinsic motivation. Computer tasks can incorporate either or both types of motivating features.

Both intrinsically and extrinsically motivated goals can influence learning behavior and outcomes, although experimental data suggest a relatively greater beneficial effect of intrinsic motivation on learning. Intrinsic motivation is associated with greater and longer-lasting learning, whereas extrinsic motivation is associated with faster but more ephemeral learning (Ryan & Deci, 2000). Therefore, intrinsically motivated students may take longer to learn the material, but they learn more and what they learn stays with them longer. Studies of educational activities that are intrinsically motivating highlight several common features: They allow for learner control, they are personalized, they are valued, and they are contextualized (Cordova & Lepper, 1996). Why should these features be intrinsically motivating? Self-determination theory posits that basic needs for autonomy, competency, and relatedness motivate people. People like to feel successful, in control, and connected to others. Accordingly, exercises that offer learner control gratify the need for autonomy, and if they are personalized, there is a greater chance for gratification of the needs for competency and relatedness. Another theory of motivation, expectancy-value theory (Wigfield & Eccles, 2000), posits that values and expectation of competency motivate people. Accordingly, exercises that are contextualized in real-life conditions will be easier to value, and activities that automatically adjust the difficulty level according to response success will keep the player feeling competent.

When a computerized cognitive activity employs instructional techniques that provide an enjoyable learning environment, contextualize learning activities in reference to real-world scenarios and personal goals, and provide opportunities for choice, emphasizing personal control and supporting self-efficacy, intrinsic motivation and learning outcomes are enhanced (Medalia & Saperstein, 2011).

## A SYSTEMATIC APPROACH TO CHOOSING COMPUTER-BASED COGNITIVE EXERCISES

Our clinical experience doing CR over the past 30 years with thousands of patients in varied treatment settings indicates that there is no one package or product that works well with everyone. Further, the products and the technology are constantly changing. We therefore recommend that the evaluation of computer-based exercises be ongoing, so that regular updates to the CR service can be made. One might start with one package and later add another or switch packages. A mixture of software and Web-based exercises can be used. Choosing appropriate programs at a programmatic level entails analyzing the many features of each program to determine which ones are appropriate remediation tools and how best to align them with the needs of a given client. There are an ever-growing number of choices available for CR, but not all programs are designed equally, and the variability in design creates distinct advantages and disadvantages for use as a CR tool and for each particular client. Box 8.1 provides a rubric for evaluating exercises, and Form 8.1 can be used to rate each activity. It is the responsibility of the therapist to evaluate and be familiar with the increasing number of programs available. This evaluation can be broken down into a series of steps and characteristics.

BOX 8.1

RUBRIC FOR REVIEWING COGNITIVE REMEDIATION TASKS

1. **Reading level required**
2. **Other prerequisite skills:** Consider computer familiarity, load on attention and working memory
3. **Cognitive deficits addressed:** Which of the following deficits are addressed?
   - Attention
   - Working memory
   - Verbal memory, visual memory
   - Problem solving, reasoning, categorization
   - Processing speed
   - Mental flexibility
   - Multi-tasking
   - Planning, prioritization, organization
4. **Adaptability of the task:**
   - There is a continuum of difficulty.
   - Level of difficulty adjusts according to accuracy of individual performance, allowing for self-pacing.
   - Hints are available.
   - Feedback is positive/negative/absent.
5. **Multimedia experience:** Is the task engaging?
   - Colorful images
   - Contextualization in a real-world activity
   - Sound effects
   - Visually interesting scenes
6. **Mediation by therapist:**
   - Ease in creating accounts for clients
   - Ease in activating and deactivating accounts
   - Ease in monitoring clients' activity (e.g., what they worked on, what level they achieved, how long they worked on a specific task)
   - Ability for the therapist to manipulate task demands (i.e., the therapist can set the level of difficulty or change other parameters of the task)
   - If the task is timed, can the timer be turned on and off?
7. **Goal properties:** Distal, proximal, specific, complex
8. **Overall strengths and weaknesses of the task:**
   - Is it interesting, fun, reinforcing?
   - Is it obvious why this task might assist clients in their everyday lives?

Name of Company and Package: _____

Name of specific activity: _____

Description of the activity: _____

**Reading level required:**

Would your clients have trouble reading it? ☐ Yes ☐ No

**Other prerequisite skills:**

☐ Little ☐ Medium ☐ Will need a lot of computer familiarity

**Cognitive deficits that can be addressed:**

☐ Attention
☐ Working memory
☐ Verbal memory
☐ Visual memory
☐ Problem solving (i.e., a circumscribed goal exists with steps needed to get there)
☐ Reasoning, categorization
☐ Processing speed
☐ Mental flexibility
☐ Multi-tasking
☐ Planning, prioritization, organization

**Adaptability of the task:**

Continuum of difficulty:

☐ Small (task does not have much range)
☐ Adequate
☐ Level of difficulty adjusts according to accuracy of individual performance

Allows for self-pacing            ☐ Yes ☐ No

Hints are available               ☐ Yes ☐ No

Feedback                          ☐ Positive ☐ Negative ☐ Absent

**Multimedia experience:**

Colorful images                   ☐ Yes ☐ No

Contextualized in a real-world activity   ☐ Yes ☐ No

Sound effects                     ☐ Yes ☐ No

Visually interesting scenes       ☐ Yes ☐ No

(continued)

**Mediation by therapist:**

Can therapist set the level of difficulty? ☐ Yes ☐ No

Can therapist change other parameters? ☐ Yes ☐ No

Is it timed? ☐ Yes ☐ No

Can timer be turned on/off? ☐ Yes ☐ No ☐ N/A

**Goal properties:**

Specific ☐ Yes ☐ No

Complex ☐ Yes ☐ No

Proximal ☐ Yes ☐ No

Distal ☐ Yes ☐ No

**Overall strengths and weaknesses:**

Is it interesting, fun, reinforcing? ☐ Yes ☐ No

*Elaborate*: _____

Is it be obvious why it might help someone in everyday life? ☐ Yes ☐ No

How might the task help someone achieve a recovery-oriented goal?

_____

# HARDWARE, SOFTWARE, AND THE INTERNET

The first step is to consider your platform, hardware, and Internet accessibility. Will the exercises be done on a computer, tablet, or phone? Next, consider the software used for CR, which can be stand-alone or Web-based. Each has its own set of benefits. Stand-alone software has the advantage of being Web-independent, making it easy to use on a laptop or a computer without Internet access, providing that the computer has a compact disc (CD) drive for titles that have not been digitized for download. Stand-alone software also has a different expense structure in that there is a one-time fee for purchase of the program, whereas the Web-based packages typically have monthly user fees. Many programs allow for multiple installations and for multiple users per installation.

Some excellent titles are several years old and available at affordable prices online. There are several titles that were developed based on learning principles and target problem solving in an appealing and contextualized virtual environment. These older activities, which include products by Edmark Corporation and Sunburst Communications as well as others, are discussed in detail in Medalia, Revheim, and Herlands (2009); they offer experiences and tasks that have not yet been replicated in Web-based programs. With age, however, come potential complications: Many older programs do not run well, or at all, because of incompatibility with current operating environments and hardware. Although adjustments can be made to Windows-based operating systems to allow them to simulate older operating environments (e.g., Windows 95), this fix is not always sufficient. As software and hardware become outdated, exercises have to be updated or retired to accommodate new platforms and systems. In addition, some newer laptops and tablet devices do not have CD drives, making installation of the older, CD-based programs impossible without the purchase of an external CD drive.

Web-based programs are proliferating and offer distinct advantages over CD-based programs. They are portable, allowing a registered user to sign in from any computer (i.e., within a clinic setting or from home). Some Web-based programs allow therapists to manage clients' accounts, monitor therapeutic activities, set assignments, and activate and deactivate user licenses. Therefore, they offer the therapist an advantage of portability as well. Further, these products are often actively updated and improved so that they will continue to run smoothly despite changes in computer hardware and the inevitable Internet browser updates. Web-based programs offer variety: Whereas CD-based programs are usually limited to a single task or a fixed number of tasks, a single Web-based package can include an ever-changing number of separate tasks. The Web platforms commonly add tasks to their packages, whereas updates to CDs usually require purchase of an upgraded product. Web-based programs also offer a variety of purchasing options, from a single-user license that may have a monthly or yearly charge to a clinic license that includes the bulk purchase of user accounts that can then be assigned to patients.

Finally, a burgeoning selection of application-based cognitive exercise pro-grams (apps) is available for smartphones and tablets. Some of these are pro-duced by the same companies that offer Web-based programs (e.g., Lumosity, Fit Brains). At present, these programs generally have fewer tasks than their Web-based cousins, as well as less user control, although this can be expected to change in time. The range of cognitive tasks offered thus far on app-based programs is largely confined to those related to processing speed, attention, visual memory, and flexibility. The format has only limited offerings for prob-lem solving (often numerically based), working memory, and auditory-based tasks in general. Interactivity is based on touch-screen responses instead of mouse-clicks and typing, and the platform appears best suited for activities involving memory and processing speed. Whereas tablets and phones offer the ultimate in portability, they are often used in noisy places or when on the go—environments that may not be conducive to attention and learning. At present, there are no app-based programs with the customizability and tracking features that are available to therapists with some of the more sophisticated Web-based programs. However, as computers and technology move more toward portable or even wearable devices (e.g., Google glass, Apple Watch, movement-tracking devices) and changes in input methods (e.g., eye tracking, motion and gesture detection), app-based programs may advance to compete and perhaps overtake their computer-based peers.

## BUDGET

Most computer-based CR exercises are found within the context of Web-based packages that are accessed by paying a monthly fee. Some companies have sev-eral packages (e.g., Posit Science, Scientific Brain Training Pro [SBTP]), whereas others offer a single package (e.g., Fit Brains, Lumosity, CIRCuiTS). Within each package are a number of cognitive training exercises, so CR therapists need to determine which packages are most likely to meet the needs of the clients they serve. When choosing a package, it is useful to consider the range of exercises offered for the monthly per-user fee and whether the exercises themselves are likely to meet client needs.

Other features also factor into the budgetary considerations. Some companies provide the option to activate and deactivate users; others do not. Given that there is often an ebb and flow of clients in a CR program, it is very helpful to have the deactivation feature. It is more expensive to purchase forty-five user memberships for the forty-five clients one expects to enroll over the course of a year than to purchase fifteen memberships for the fifteen clients that are likely to be enrolled at any given time.

Another feature to consider is whether there are administration and monitoring tools for the clinician (e.g., BrainHQ, Cogmed, SBTP) or only single-user licenses (e.g., Fit Brains, Lumosity). For a therapist who assigns homework or allows patients to access CR exercises independently or from home, having access to monitoring tools such as those embedded in Cogmed or SBTP can be very useful. The monitoring tools allow the therapist to observe the exercises used, the duration of time on task, and the level achieved on task. Not only can the therapist ensure compliance, but he or she can use the data gathered to guide interventions. For example, if the therapist observes that the patient is spending a relatively short time on a particular task or avoids it completely for several usage days, the therapist can work with the patient to identify the nature of the difficulty. The task may be too difficult or too easy, leading to frustration or boredom, respectively. The patient may question the utility of the task and may need the therapist to bridge the task to the individual's goals. Sometimes, the issue is software malfunction or "glitches" that prevent the task from operating properly. The administrative and monitoring tools can shed light on the issues underlying a patient's difficulty performing recommended exercises.

The other way in which cognitive exercises are obtained is by purchasing software or finding specific Web-based exercises. Software is usually sold for use on a specific number (e.g., one, two to five) or sometimes an unlimited number of computers, and an unlimited number of people can use it at the designated computers. Specific Web-based exercises are also available and can be purchased or sometimes accessed for free.

## LANGUAGE REQUIREMENTS

When considering software, it is important to notice the reading level required for the program and the degree to which language, vocabulary, and reading are required to utilize the program. This is important not only for non–English-speaking clients but for clients with dyslexia, poor visual acuity, low IQ, low educational level, or markedly impaired sustained attention, for whom lengthy written instructions will be poorly understood. Software programs developed by educational companies usually indicate on the packaging the required reading level or the intended grade (e.g., K-5, 6-8, 9-12). This designation relates to the intellectual sophistication of the program, the language requirements, and the general maturity level of the games. For example, some of the games with younger intended target audiences have a distinctly cartoonish quality, which some clients may not tolerate or may feel is infantilizing. Many of the Web-based programs do not indicate a minimum reading level, so the therapist should evaluate each task to determine how much reading is required in the instructions and whether the task is language based. For language-based tasks, it is important to notice whether the stimuli are presented in written or auditory form and how that aligns with an individual client's abilities and needs. Some programs are translated from the culture and language of origin in ways that may not be wholly culturally and regionally compatible, making for odd word choices or use of language.

## TARGETED COGNITIVE SKILLS

CR software packages differ in the range of cognitive skills that are trained. If cognitive skills are considered as existing on a hierarchy, then basic sensory processing would be at the bottom of the hierarchy and problem solving—the most synthetic skill—would be toward the top of the hierarchy. From this perspective, the processing of auditory sounds is a more basic skill than the memorization of words, and identifying the similarities among words (e.g., apple, plum, and orange are all fruits) is a more complex task than remembering words.

One approach to CR proceeds by training the more basic cognitive skills first and slowly working up to the more complex skills; another approach (called "top down") assumes that by training a complex skill such as problem solving, the component skills will also be addressed. At this juncture, there is no definitive research supporting one approach over the other, and indeed the meta-analytic studies suggest that both approaches are efficacious (Wykes, Huddy, Cellard, McGurk, & Czobor, 2011). However, these different theoretical orientations influence the range and type of cognitive exercises that are offered. Some companies focus on providing exercises at the bottom of the hierarchy, others provide exercises in the middle range, and some focus on the higher-order cognitive skills. For example, at Posit Science, the scientific advisory team wants exercises that address deficits in basic sensory processing, because those are seen as underlying cognitive impairments in higher-order cognitive skills such as memory. Accordingly, that company emphasizes the importance of training basic sensory skills such as auditory tone discrimination, and they offer fewer problem-solving exercises than might be found in other packages. At other companies, such as Lumosity and SBTP, there is little emphasis on training sensory processing, and the range of exercises includes a focus on problem solving. Cogmed has three packages that all focus exclusively on working memory exercises.

In evaluating software, the therapist should consider whether a particular program offers a range of tasks that reflect an understanding of cognition on a hierarchy and, if so, how broad that hierarchy is. Further, is there user choice, or does the program automatically move the user through a prescribed hierarchy of exercises? Posit Science, for example, has one package called Brain Fitness, which automatically moves the user through a hierarchy of tasks from basic sensory processing to verbal memory with minimal option for user choice, and a different package which offers exercises that train basic visual and auditory sensory processing with the user able to choose whether or not to play them.

With some software, users can view visual "sweeps," in which they must distinguish and identify the orientation and movement of a series of lines that are presented at progressively faster speeds. The auditory equivalent here asks users to detect changes in the pitch of sounds. In addition to these low-level basic sensory processing tasks, BrainHQ offers other tasks that provide increasing complexity, requiring the integration of multiple cognitive skills in the performance of the exercise. Still, the user and the therapist are offered choice as to the sequence of presentation; the tasks are not presented in a forced, hierarchical order.

Fit Brains approaches training somewhat differently. Two versions of their program are offered, the current version and the "classic" version. The current version offers tasks that are designed to train specific, fairly discrete cognitive skills, although it does not offer the most basic level of sensory processing as BrainHQ does. The classic version provides activities that train skills on tasks requiring the activation of multiple cognitive skills simultaneously (e.g., requiring visual scanning, reading, inferential reasoning, working memory, and visual memory on a single task). Lumosity and SBTP allow for user choice in accessing tasks on the hierarchy, and although basic sensory processing is not included, there are numerous exercises that vary in the degree to which discrete or complex/multiple cognitive skills are utilized.

## EDUCATIONAL AND MOTIVATIONAL FACTORS

Educational research has revealed several factors that promote intrinsic motivation, learning, and engagement in tasks. These factors are critical to consider in CR because clients who are engaged and motivated are more likely to attend sessions, participate in the activities, remain in treatment for longer periods of time, and engage in the treatment more deeply (Medalia & Saperstein, 2013). The result is that motivated and engaged clients will see maximal improvements and will benefit most from treatment. It is therefore clinically advisable to utilize programs that incorporate educational and motivational enhancements such as sensory appeal, personalization, contextualization, user control, goal properties, feedback and positive reinforcement, dynamic level adjustment, and range of difficulty. Each of these characteristics is defined and described in detail in the following sections.

### Sensory Appeal and Perception

Sensory appeal and perceptual requirements refer to the visual and auditory experience of the user when interacting with the program and the degree to which accurate gameplay is dependent on perception. Visual appeal refers to the visual design characteristics of the program. Specifically, the therapist should consider the degree to which the visual experience is interesting and stimulating. Consider the game environment: Is it colorful or bland? Is the visual experience appealing and interesting? Does the environment change, or is it static? Notice whether gameplay is dependent on color discrimination (important to consider for patients with color blindness). Similarly, are sounds used to enhance or detract from the user's experience? Is the user treated to rewarding sounds for correct responses, and is there background music? Can the user choose or make adjustments to the type and volume of background music? If a program has digitized speaking, is it clear and well articulated?

## Personalization

Educators and video game makers have long known that users enjoy personalization. It enhances learning and depth of engagement in a task (Cordova & Lepper, 1996; Graesser et al., 2008). Personalization can be as simple as logging on with one's username; other examples are customizing the environment (e.g., changing the background and colors, adding personal touches to one's email signature) and creating whole characters and assigning characteristics to aspects of the game or activity. Personalization also refers to how well the exercise suits the user's learning style and cognitive deficits and to what degree the program does this via built-in assessment, rather than relying on therapist input of exercise features to customize the learning experience.

Personalization can be evident in the capacity of the program to adjust the level of difficulty based on the person's performance or to provide an appropriate range of practice opportunities given the person's level of functioning. Software programs often use task performance to automatically adjust the level of difficulty. Some programs require the user to complete an assessment before beginning a task so that an appropriate starting level can be provided. Others begin all users at the easiest levels, requiring a certain level of performance to earn a promotion to the next level. Many software programs use an algorithm to achieve maximal engagement in a cognitive activity by maintaining the level of difficulty at an 80% success rate so that learners are continuously challenged while frustration is minimized. Personalization of the difficulty level has the advantage of promoting a sense of competency, which in turn keeps the user engaged in the learning task. Perceived competency for learning tasks is a strong predictor of both staying motivated to learn and actually making cognitive gains. People with schizophrenia who anticipate being competent on learning tasks tend to choose more difficult tasks, persist more, and achieve a higher level of success (Choi, Fiszdon, & Medalia, 2010).

## Contextualization

Another important dimension on which to consider tasks is contextualization. Simply put, is the cognitive exercise embedded in an activity or atmosphere that is reminiscent or representative of a real-world task or situation? For example, a computational task to aid working memory could be presented as an auditory or visual set of numbers that must be serially added mentally over a specified span of time. This would be an example of a decontextualized working memory task utilizing numbers. Alternatively, this same task could be embedded in a virtual grocery store where the user is tasked with being the cashier whose register broke—now we have a working memory task placed in context. The context is a grocery store, and the user is simulating work as a grocery store cashier.

There are distinct advantages to contextualized learning for promoting motivation and generalization. A contextualized task allows users to more readily recognize the value of the task and how it might relate to their overall goal. For example, remembering names and faces is readily valued as useful in a variety of contexts (e.g., social gatherings, work), whereas learning increasingly longer lists of random words is a less common everyday task. When the task value is readily appreciated, there is increased interest, effort, engagement, learning, and intrinsic motivation. Contextualization also facilitates generalization, which, as discussed earlier, is the process by which a skill trained in one context is able to be applied broadly. The context becomes the cue that activates use of the cognitive skill. For example, after working on an attention task that is contextualized as a road trip, the person learns to activate attention processes when traveling.

Contextualization requires sensitivity to cultural and demographic factors. Cogmed is an example of a company that has manipulated the contextualization of their tasks in order to accommodate the different learning needs of preschool children, school-aged children, and adults. Younger children respond to more fanciful contexts, whereas adults may appreciate a context that more closely resembles the real world.

## User Control

As mentioned previously, intrinsic motivation is key for learning to be lasting. One way in which intrinsic motivation can be facilitated is by providing opportunities for autonomous learning (as explained in self-determination theory). User control is a key factor in creating a sense of autonomy. Many tasks provide an opportunity for learner control by giving choice; when people are allowed to have a choice about their learning experience, they feel in more control (Cordova & Lepper, 1996; Ryan & Deci, 2000).

There are a variety of ways in which exercises can provide opportunities for learner control. The programs vary in the extent to which they are restrictive or easily directed by the user. For example, some Web-based and smartphone-based apps prescribe a set of daily activities. There is no user control in the choice of activities, the duration for which each is played, the characteristics of the particular activities, or their sequence. Although this set-up may provide for a nice variety and perhaps a hierarchy of skills, it is entirely predetermined. This poses a risk to a poorly or moderately intrinsically motivated user, who may lose interest or willingness to engage in a CR activity that is too challenging or is considered boring, particularly if such tasks appear early in the predetermined sequence. Conversely, this same user would be more likely to engage in tasks—even those that are challenging or less appealing—if allowed to choose the sequence and duration of the activities. Further, with sequence flexibility, the therapist could help guide the user in choosing the order of activities, with the aim of increasing a sense of competence. Choosing activities in which the user is likely to meet success early in the sequence and placing the more challenging or potentially frustrating activities later in the order allows the user to develop greater resilience and frustration tolerance.

## Goal Properties

The nature of a client's goals can have a large impact on motivation. If it takes many steps to reach a goal, there are more chances to lose motivation, and if a goal is complex, it can be difficult to identify when one is near completion. Tasks that require only one activity (e.g., sort the laundry by color) and a set number of repetitions have goal properties that are specific and proximal. Tasks that require multiple steps (e.g., make a three-course dinner) have more complex and distal goals. Some tasks are well defined (e.g., do three math problems), whereas others have a less defined completion point (e.g., study for an examination). People with poor attention and working memory can have difficulty with tasks that have distal and complex goals, yet those are the types of tasks that are commonly found in real-life situations.

In CR programs, it can be helpful to have tasks with a range of goal properties so that people can start out with tasks that have specific, proximal goals. Then, as working memory and attention improve, they can move to tasks with more complex and distal goals. There is a range of goal properties that can be found on CR Web-based packages, although many tend to be more proximal and specific than is characteristic of the tasks required in everyday life. When considering the goal properties of a task, an important consideration is whether it has properties common to the types of tasks the user will face in everyday life.

## Feedback and Reinforcement

Feedback has the potential to be motivating or demotivating, affecting whether a person is willing to continue on a specific exercise or in the overall CR program. Considerable research has been done within the field of education to identify what kinds of feedback are likely to motivate a person in the learning context (Schunk & Zimmerman, 2008). Specific, goal-oriented feedback from a credible source, delivered within and after the completion of a task, helps to shape behavior and provides encouragement to stay on task. Feedback provides information to users about their performance, their progress, and their overall skill relative to others. Well-placed feedback within tasks (i.e., immediately after a response) helps users to learn—either to replicate a response or technique or to try a different approach. The more immediate and salient the feedback, the more likely it is that users will notice and make use of the feedback to shape their behavior. This is especially important for users with psychotic disorders, who may perseverate and may take longer to respond to environmental feedback with changes in their behavior.

Clinicians who are evaluating computerized CR tasks should note the presence and quality of the feedback. Within the task, are there rewarding sounds, a spoken "Way to go!," or a written message indicating "Good work"? What happens if the user makes a mistake? Does the computer activity make strong negative comments such as "You failed"? Notice how the overall task is structured. Is it divided into levels, and are the levels arranged hierarchically? Are the differences in degree of difficulty from level-to-level articulated to the user? In other words, does the feedback help the user both appreciate the challenge ahead and perceive what has been mastered on previous levels?

Another kind of feedback orients the participant to the utility value of the task. *Utility value* refers to how important the user ranks the task or cognitive skill in relation to his or her individual goals. Utility value is easier to appreciate when cognitive or task challenges are discussed in real-world terms. For example, feedback on a divided attention task might be read as follows: "Good progress. You can also use these divided attention skills when you are talking to several friends at once." Tasks with a high perceived utility value result in a higher level of engagement and higher intrinsic motivation (Wigfield & Eccles, 2000). This is seen in the example of a user whose goal is to improve her performance as a receptionist, and specifically to improve her memory for what she hears. This user would likely consider an auditory memory task as having a high utility value, because she would consider improvements in auditory memory as having a direct impact on her job-related goal.

Examples of educational software that provides in-task reinforcement and feedback include titles such as *Thinking Things* (Edmark) and *Factory Deluxe* (Sunburst). They provide direct reinforcement for correct responses as well as supportive feedback for incorrect responses, such as "Try again" or "Keep trying." These programs also use a hierarchy of difficulty, indicated by levels (1, 2, 3 or A, B, C) and, in some cases, by descriptions of the challenge inherent in each level. BrainHQ is a Web-based program that provides auditory feedback for successful trials as well as visual displays of real-time, in-task improvements. It also provides evaluative data after each task is completed, usually in the form of starting and ending speeds and number of stars achieved. However, there is no explanation of the star system, which may leave users wondering about the utility value of their performance level and of the task in general. BrainHQ does set up the levels in a hierarchy of difficulty along two axes and provides a basic description of the characteristic of the task. The tasks become more complex as one unlocks levels along each axis.

SBTP has hierarchical levels and specifies for the user the criteria for success and advancement to the next level. Within tasks, not much positive reinforcement is offered, but many of the tasks allow for a review of correct and incorrect responses at the end of the task. This provides valuable information to users about the quality of their performance and areas that are in need of improvement and focus in a subsequent round.

There may be variability in the feedback provided on various tasks within any given package of exercises, so the clinician needs to consider how feedback is handled generally across exercises in the package. There is also a wide variety of styles in feedback and performance evaluation among the available commercial cognitive enhancement programs. Fit Brains has minimal in-exercise feedback but does provide clear information at the conclusion of an exercise regarding the percentage of correct responses and whether the performance was sufficient to unlock the next level. Lumosity provides checks and x's as well as tones within the exercise to signal correct and incorrect responses, as well as a numerical score, number of trials correct, and percentage correct score at the end. Different still is BrainHQ, which provides a numerical description of the current performance (often giving the maximum speed of correct responding in milliseconds) and grades the performance on a five-star scale. The programs also differ in the ways in which they provide summary data to users. Both BrainHQ and Lumosity, for example, provide detailed overall performance summary pages ("Progress" and "Brain Profile," respectively) that represent in percentile rank the user's overall cognitive performance and performance on specific cognitive skills compared with the performance of other same-aged participants who use the program. Fit Brains provides the same type of feedback by representing a user's performance in terms of the "percentage of same-aged users who are stronger than you in each area." Each program has unique graphical presentations of the data and proprietary metrics such as the "Lumosity Performance Index" and the "Fit Brains Index."

The wide variety of styles in feedback and performance evaluation among the available cognitive enhancement programs can be confusing to clients. Therefore, when evaluating and using software, it is important to consider the experience provided for the client in terms of positive reinforcement and clarity in the feedback. It is helpful for the therapist to be familiar with the type and style of feedback provided and to supplement and provide explanations as needed for each client to maximize motivation, learning, and generalization.

## Ceilings, Floors, and Dynamic Titration

Cognitive abilities fluctuate. This is true for the general population, and it is true for patients undergoing CR. Variation can be caused by simple changes in sleep or general health or by fluctuations in mental health, such as a psychotic episode or an acute depressive episode. In short, recovery is not always linear, and patients may have ups and downs in their cognitive performance. The available CR programs handle this intrapersonal variation in different ways. Those games that titrate difficulty within a chosen level dynamically (i.e., either up or down based on the user's performance) are best able to maintain an optimal difficulty level. Cogmed and BrainHQ are examples of packages that provide this type of user experience. In Brain HQ, after three consecutive errors (indicated to the user by a tone and a red mark on the progress bar above the activity), the difficulty level steps down. Programs that do not have this feature do not respond to repeated failed efforts on a given level by making the activity easier or demoting the user to an earlier level; they simply advance the person if a certain score is achieved.

Therefore, a patient who once achieved a high level on an activity but later returns to the exercise performing less well will be offered only that previously achieved high level of difficulty, however many failed attempts are made. Without the intervention of the therapist, the outcome will be negative.

BrainHQ provides an example of real-time dynamic adjustments in level of difficulty as well as manual adjustment of the level in which to work (level 1, 2, or 3). Other programs also allow for therapist adjustment of the user experience. Fit Brains and Fit Brains Classic allow for the selection of Beginner, Intermediate, or Advanced level at the start of an exercise once all levels have been unlocked. Therefore, rather than allowing a user who is struggling with a task on a particular day work to frustration at an advanced level, the therapist could intervene and suggest moving to a lower level to achieve success on the task.

Many of the CD-based games have levels through which a user can progress, but rarely do they automatically titrate to a lower level of difficulty with repeated failures. However, most do allow for the user or therapist to manually move the user to a lower level. *Thinking Things 3*, for example, moves the user up with successive achievements at a given level, but any level can be easily accessed and selected manually, and the task demands and challenges at each level are indicated, allowing the therapist to position the user at the ideal level on any given day.

The capacity of computer programs to offer dynamic titration impacts the role of the therapist conducting the CR sessions. Will the therapist need to guide the patient to an easier level if the task as a whole is proving too challenging (i.e., too many failures) or the patient becomes frustrated (evident in verbalizations or behaviors reflective of frustration or loss of confidence)? In that case, the therapist may also need to normalize and explain the difficulty the patient is having and the rationale for moving the activity to an easier level or putting the entire exercise aside for a time. Without such interventions from the therapist, the patient may feel defeated, may lose the sense of competence, and may even begin to doubt the efficacy of CR. Failures and frustrations need to be dealt with promptly and skillfully to mitigate the longer-term negative effects of such an experience, particularly with less-engaged patients and patients who are just beginning this work.

## THE ROLE OF TECHNOLOGICAL ADVANCEMENT

The rapid pace of change in technology means that products are frequently changing or being added to the marketplace. Companies take different approaches to upgrading and expanding their product lines: Some constantly add new exercises to their portfolio, and others do so at a slower pace. Some companies are eager for feedback from clinicians and clients and update their products accordingly, whereas others are less interactive with their consumers. It can be safely assumed that the products available to purchase now will be quite different 2 years from now. We therefore recommend that product evaluation be an ongoing activity and that budget planning assume additions and deletions in the computer-based exercises that are purchased. Dedicated time to review new products and examine client satisfaction with the currently used products can be built into the job description of the CR therapist. This ensures that the materials used will be current and optimal for promoting cognitive health.

Research can play an important role in product expansion. A certain level of user confidence is accorded when an exercise has been used successfully in randomized controlled trials. However, exclusive reliance on randomized controlled trials to recommend an exercise or package would disregard the fact that clinical services are typically quite different from research environments. It takes years for research to be completed, and the products may be technologically inferior by that time. The other way to find products is to have a systematic approach to evaluating cognitive exercises, one that is grounded in theory, research, and clinical practice. That is the approach offered in this chapter.

## SUMMARY

Computerized cognitive exercises are a central feature of most restorative CR programs, and the clinician faces challenging decisions when choosing activities. Because no one selection will work in all settings or for all patients, there is a need for different products. Fortunately, there are many products to choose from. This chapter has reviewed the many factors to consider so that exercises will be appropriate to the program and to all the patients' needs.

## REFERENCES

Choi J., Fiszdon, J. M., & Medalia, A. (2010). Expectancy-value theory in persistence of learning effects in schizophrenia: Role of task value and perceived competency *Schizophrenia Bulletin, 36*, 957–965.

Choi, J., & Medalia, A. (2010). Intrinsic motivation and learning in a schizophrenia spectrum sample. *Schizophrenia Research, 118*, 12–19.

Cordova, D. I., & Lepper, M. R. (1996). Intrinsic motivation and the process of learning: Beneficial effects of contextualization, personalization, and choice. *Journal of Educational Psychology, 88*, 715–730.

Graesser, A. C., Jeon, M., & Dufty, D. (2008) Agent technologies designed to facilitate interactive knowledge construction. *Discourse Processes, 45*, 298–322.

Medalia, A., Revheim, N., & Herlands, T. (2009). *Cognitive remediation for psychological disorders, therapist guide*. Treatments That Work series. New York, NY: Oxford University Press.

Medalia, A., & Saperstein, A. (2011). The role of motivation for treatment success. *Schizophrenia Bulletin, 37*, 122–128.

Medalia, A., & Saperstein, A. M. (2013). Does cognitive remediation for schizophrenia improve functional outcomes? *Current Opinion in Psychiatry, 26*, 151–157.

Ryan, R. M., & Deci, E. L. (2000). Self-determination theory and the facilitation of intrinsic motivation, social development, and well-being. *The American Psychologist, 55*, 68–78.

Schunk, D. H., & Zimmerman, B. J. (2008). *Motivation and self-regulated learning: Theory, research, and applications.* New Jersey: Erlbaum.

Shepard, R. N. (1987). Toward a universal law of generalization for psychological science. *Science, 237,* 1317–1323.

Wigfield, A., & Eccles, J. (2000). Expectancy-value theory of achievement motivation. *Contemporary Educational Psychology, 25,* 68–81.

Wykes, T., Huddy, V., Cellard, C., McGurk, S. R., & Czobor, P. (2011). A meta-analysis of cognitive remediation for schizophrenia: Methodology and effect sizes. *The American Journal of Psychiatry,168,* 472–485.

# 9

# Compensatory Approaches to Improving Functioning

ELIZABETH W. TWAMLEY ■

## INTRODUCTION

Due in large part to cognitive impairments, people with psychiatric illnesses often have difficulty with everyday activities, including self-care and living independently, succeeding at school or work, and initiating and maintaining meaningful social and romantic relationships (Green, 1996; Heinrichs & Zakzanis, 1998; McGurk & Mueser, 2004; Palmer et al., 2002; Twamley et al., 2002). Having a psychiatric illness often results in fewer brain resources being available for paying attention, learning new information, or solving problems. Deficits in areas such as attention, learning, and executive functioning have repeatedly been shown to negatively affect real-world outcomes (Green & Nuechterlein, 1999; Twamley et al., 2003). Improving functioning in these domains requires the use of cognitive skills and strategies that many healthy people use on a daily basis. Functioning can also be enhanced by structuring the environment to maximally support activities in these domains.

The purpose of any rehabilitation intervention is to enable a person with a disability to achieve an optimal level of performance and quality of life by reducing the impact of the disability on daily activities. Reducing the deficit or impairment directly is one potential route to improving functioning; working around the deficit or impairment and participating in activities or completing life tasks in new or different ways is another way of reducing disability. This chapter discusses compensatory cognitive strategies and environmental modifications that can be helpful in improving performance of everyday activities needed for successful functioning at home, school, and work and in relationships. Compensatory interventions and environmental modifications can help people bypass or compensate for their cognitive impairments. The goals of such interventions are to reduce cognitive demands in the environment, conserve cognitive energy for more complex tasks, and bypass cognitive impairments by using routines or compensatory strategies when approaching tasks.

Compensatory cognitive strategies are tools to work around impairments in cognitive domains such as attention, learning, and executive functioning. They do not promise to restore functioning to the way it was before illness onset or to a "normal" state. Cognitive compensations (e.g., smartphones, electronic calendars, to-do lists) are used by many successful people and are increasingly acceptable to people with cognitive impairments in the mobile device era. There are Web sites devoted to helping people with cognitive challenges learn to use mobile devices (e.g., smartphones, tablets) while simultaneously drawing parallels to the cognitive skills underlying these technical skills (see, for example, http://id4theweb.com/). There are also reviews of mobile applications that are especially helpful for users with cognitive impairments (http://id4theweb.com/appreviews/). Compensatory strategies are consistent with the positive psychology approach (Duckworth, Steen, & Seligman, 2005), which emphasizes the use of strengths to accomplish goals rather than focusing on deficits. As with all behavioral and psychotherapeutic interventions, the goal of compensatory cognitive training is for the strategies learned in session to be strengthened into habits used in the real world and for therapeutic gains to generalize to meaningful real-world outcomes.

Linking strategies to personally meaningful functional goals improves the likelihood that goal-related strategies will generalize to meaningful real-world outcomes (Granholm, Holden, Link, & McQuaid, 2014). When therapists plan for generalization from the beginning and use real-world activities as much as possible, the path between strategy practice and real-world implementation is shorter, and the chance of generalization improves dramatically. Use of individualized goals also increases client "buy-in," as does use of real-world activities that are meaningful to the client. When clients experience success in activities that are meaningful to them, they may feel encouraged to try more new activities rather than avoiding activities that are viewed as cognitively demanding or difficult.

Sometimes, clients (and therapists!) get so focused on practicing cognitive strategies that they lose sight of the big picture and forget why they are practicing the strategies in the first place. Consistently linking the strategies with the client's individualized goals helps both the client and the therapist stay on track, thereby bridging the "skill-goal gap." This can be done by (a) introducing the strategy to be taught, (b) reminding the client of his or her stated goals, (c) linking the strategies to be learned to specific goals, and (d) eliciting agreement that the strategies will be important for reaching the stated goals. For example, the therapist may say,

> We are going to practice some strategies today that will help you pay attention during conversations. You told me that you want to get a job and start dating again. To get a job, you will need to pay attention during a job interview, and once you get the job, you'll have to pay attention during conversations with your supervisor and co-workers. You might have to have a conversation to get a first date, and you'll need to be able to focus on conversations on that first date in order to get a second date. Would you agree that improving your

focus during conversations is a good way to work toward your ultimate goals of getting a job and going on dates?

Environmental modification interventions attempt to reduce the cognitive demands in the individual's environment to improve functioning. Examples of environmental modifications include use of electronic or paper reminders in the home, organization and planning of clothing to wear for the week, and use of devices such as pillboxes and alarm clocks (Velligan et al., 2002). Typically, these approaches require a therapist who helps clients modify their surroundings to simplify and routinize daily activities. These environmental approaches can be very effective because they are home based and include personally relevant, easily implemented changes to the client's surroundings, but therapist involvement may be extensive and long-term (Kidd et al., 2014). Additionally, gains in functioning at home may not generalize to other environments.

Compensatory or environmental strategies can be used as stand-alone interventions or combined with restorative approaches discussed in other chapters in this volume. Compelling evidence now exists to show that participants treated with restorative interventions can show cognitive improvement, and meta-analyses indicate that restorative interventions can have additional effects on real-world functioning when they are paired with strategy coaching or compensatory training (McGurk, Twamley, Sitzer, McHugo, & Mueser, 2007; Wykes, Huddy, Cellard, McGurk, & Czobor, 2011). Thus, combining computerized or other restorative cognitive training programs with compensatory cognitive training may result in the most improvement in real-world functioning.

## COMPENSATORY COGNITIVE TRAINING

Compensatory Cognitive Training, or CCT (Twamley, Burton, & Vella, 2011; Twamley, Vella, Burton, Heaton, & Jeste, 2012) is an approach that combines compensatory strategy training with client-driven environmental modifications; the objective is an intervention that is brief, low-tech, low-cost, portable, practical, and generalizable to a wide variety of real-world situations. The goal of the intervention is to help clients learn and develop cognitive strategies to form long-term habits that are meaningful in the real world. Habit learning has several advantages: It is more similar to procedural learning (i.e., learning the steps of an action such as tying one's shoes) than to declarative memory (i.e., memory for facts and information) (Bayley, Frascino, & Squire, 2005; Knowlton, Mangels, & Squire, 1996); it is intact in people with psychiatric illness (Clare, McKenna, Mortimer, & Baddeley, 1993; Keri et al., 2005); and it is resistant to forgetting (Bayley et al., 2005).

The *Compensatory Cognitive Training Manual* (client and therapist versions are available free of charge at www.cogsmart.com) presents a twelve-session curriculum that is designed to be administered individually (about 1 hour per week for 12 weeks) or in groups of four to eight (about 2 hours per week for 12 weeks).

There are advantages to both individual and group approaches. Working on an individual basis allows the clinician to tailor the CCT curriculum to the client, moving more quickly through some concepts and spending a longer time on others. Working with groups allows for a more structured, classroom-type experience that is particularly attractive to some clients, and it also allows for group support in learning and applying the strategies. Some clients are more willing to try something new if they see another person experience success. Regardless of whether it is administered individually or in a group, it can be called a "cognitive training class" rather than a "group" or "therapy" to emphasize the skill-based nature of the intervention and to reduce stigma. Masters-level or doctoral-level mental health clinicians are typically well prepared to provide CCT, and tips are provided on the back-facing pages of the therapist version of the manual so that clinicians who have never provided cognitive training before will feel confident and prepared.

Although CCT is a brief intervention, 12 weeks is typically enough time for clients to practice strategies and consolidate new cognitive habits. Strategies are practiced through interactive, game-like activities to maintain interest and increase focus and motivation; clients' personal goals are elicited to enhance intrinsic motivation and foster sustained attendance (Choi & Medalia, 2005). Client goals typically fall into one of six domains: living situation, school, work, social relationships, finances, or health. Clients write about their goals during the first session of the intervention (Form 9.1) and revisit their goals frequently in order to bridge the "skill-goal gap" and increase motivation to practice their strategies in the community. Many real-world examples of how strategy use can be helpful are provided. For example,

- Using a calendar efficiently will help you plan your job search activities or work/school assignments, go to work or class on time, call your best friend on his birthday, pay the rent on time, and generally get things done.
- Using conversational attention skills will help your relationships with your family members, friends, partners, or bosses by making sure that other people feel heard and understood; these skills will also help you remember your conversations better.
- Learning and memory strategies can help you learn and remember new information at home, work, and school.
- Executive functioning strategies can help you with planning, prioritizing, problem-solving, and thinking flexibly. These skills are important in managing your tasks in life, whether they involve work, school, relationships, health, finances, or living independently.

Some clients have difficulty coming up with concrete goals but express dissatisfaction with their living situation, learning or educational status, work situation, social life, health, or financial situation. Exploring their dissatisfaction can lead to the formation of individual goals.

**Think about your goals for the course:**

1.  What are one or two **problems with cognition or thinking** that affect you most (e.g., problems remembering things, focusing, poor organization)?

    _____

    _____

    _____

2.  What **important life areas do these problems interfere with** the most (e.g., work, family relationships, managing your affairs, taking care of your health)?

    _____

    _____

    _____

3.  Identify one or two **important life goals** you would like to work toward during this course (e.g., returning to work or school, being more reliable at work, helping out more at home, remembering medications and appointments).

    _____

    _____

    _____

It is also recommended that family members or other support people be involved as much as possible. Loved ones can be powerful allies in treatment and can benefit from education regarding the client's cognitive challenges and the strategies taught in CCT. The more others know about the strategies, the more they can reinforce the client's strategy use in the real world. Helping both clients and their family members understand the cognitive challenges that often accompany psychiatric illness is an important part of treatment. A comprehensive guide for families and friends has been published by the New York State Office of Mental Health (Medalia & Revheim, 2002) and may be downloaded from http://www.omh.ny.gov/omhweb/cogdys_manual/CogDysHndbk.pdf.

Home exercises are assigned at the end of each session. They are designed to promote strategy use in the real world and to provide an opportunity to troubleshoot barriers or difficulties that arise. An example of a home exercise assignment page is presented in Form 9.2. Each session includes a review of the home exercise and previous strategies, then focuses on introducing and practicing new compensatory strategies and developing individualized plans to implement the strategies in daily life.

The CCT manual incorporates ideas and materials from various sources, including the Acquired Brain Injury program at Mesa College in San Diego (calendar training and to-do lists), the social skills training manual published in 1997 by Bellack, Mueser, Gingerich, and Agresta (conversational vigilance skills, six-step problem-solving method), Meichenbaum and Cameron's (1973) work on self-talk for task vigilance, and Delahunty and Morice's (1993) manual (also used by Wykes, Reeder, Corner, Williams, & Everitt,1999) for categorization tasks. Clients are encouraged to practice and master the strategies taught so they are able to use them automatically when the need arises. They are also encouraged to think of the strategies like a toolbox; they may use some tools frequently and some only occasionally, but it makes sense to learn how to use all the tools.

The cognitive strategies that are taught and practiced in CCT target four neuropsychological domains: prospective memory, attention and vigilance, learning and memory, and executive functioning. These domains were selected based on their importance for real-world functioning and their modifiability (Green, 1996; Green & Nuechterlein, 1999; Twamley et al., 2003). Key strategies in each domain are discussed in the following sections and summarized in Table 9.1.

## PROSPECTIVE MEMORY

The first three CCT sessions focus on prospective memory (i.e., remembering to remember), the cornerstone strategy being daily calendar use. Paper calendars are provided to all clients so that they can start using them immediately, and a variety of calendar sizes and formats are offered to ensure that clients will be able to carry their calendars everywhere they go. However, clients who have smartphones and want to use their smartphone's calendar application are encouraged to do so. Clients are encouraged to check their calendar daily or more often, as needed,

### Session 1: Home Exercise

☐ Make a "Home" for your most important personal items (e.g., calendar, keys, wallet, cellphone).
1. Choose a container.
   a. It might be a large bowl, a small box, or a backpack.
   b. If using a backpack, designate one section or pocket just for personal items only.
2. Decide **where** the container will be kept in your home.
   a. It might be on a table near the front door, on a table near the coat closet, or on a desk in the office or kitchen.
   b. It should be a convenient location that you will easily get into the habit of using every time you enter your home.
3. Start using this **"Home"** for your personal items **every day**.

☐ Carry your calendar with you every day. Enter all the upcoming doctor appointments or other activities that you know about, including this course.

☐ Decide how you will remember to bring your binder and calendar to the next session.
1. Some examples:
   a. You could put your binder in the **"Home"** you created.
   b. You could put a **sticky note** on your front door.
   c. You could ask a **significant other** or housemate to remind you.

2. Briefly **describe** how you will remember these items each session:

_____

_____

_____

*Table 9.1.* Key Domains and Strategies Included in Compensatory Cognitive Training

| Cognitive Domain | Key Strategies Taught |
|---|---|
| Prospective memory | Calendar use, to-do lists, prioritizing tasks, linking tasks by using planned cues, automatic places, using routines to automate tasks |
| Attention and vigilance | Eye contact, paraphrasing, and asking questions during conversations; self-talk during tasks; taking breaks to refocus |
| Learning and memory | Taking notes, association, chunking, categorization, acronyms, visual imagery, overlearning |
| Executive functioning | Six-step problem-solving method, self-talk and self-monitoring while solving problems, hypothesis testing using pro and con evidence, set shifting, set maintenance |

and to have a planning session once a week to add new appointments and review the week ahead. Calendar entries are reviewed regularly to monitor and optimize the amount of detail; clients must include enough detail for the calendar entry to make sense while omitting unnecessary details. Clients are also taught how to create to-do lists and how to incorporate them into their calendar (e.g., using sticky notes that can be moved from week to week, using a smartphone application for notes or reminders). The technique of linking tasks together is also taught to help clients remember to do an activity by pairing it with an activity they already do automatically (e.g., taking medication right after brushing your teeth). It can be difficult for clients to remember to check their calendars every day, so linking tasks is used to form the habit of daily calendar checking (e.g., check calendar while drinking morning coffee or before getting dressed for the day). Alarms in clocks or within smartphones are also used as cues to check the calendar or complete other daily tasks such as taking medications, attending appointments, or performing work or school assignments.

The use of "can't-miss reminders" is another important prospective memory strategy. Placing reminders where the client will be sure to see them increases the probability of accomplishing the desired task. Written reminders should preferably be placed on something the client is sure to touch during the day, because touching the reminder increases attention to its content; a sea of sticky notes on a refrigerator, bathroom mirror, or computer monitor will quickly blend into the background and be overlooked, but a reminder that needs to be touched (e.g., on a doorknob or faucet handle) is less likely to be ignored. Any reminders that will be easily seen or heard are desirable, such as reminders that are written on one's hand, left as a voicemail, or even sent as a text or email to oneself. General strategies for organization around the home, such as always keeping important objects (wallet, keys, phone, pillbox) in an "automatic place," also enhance prospective memory by making these items visible and encouraging routine, in addition to preventing the items from being misplaced.

## ATTENTION AND VIGILANCE

The next sessions target conversational and task vigilance to help clients maintain focus and improve attention during conversations and while working on tasks. The conversational vigilance content uses the acronym LEAP (Fig. 9.1) to describe four "golden rules" of paying attention during conversations: (a) Listen actively (e.g., make eye contact); (b) Eliminate distractions in the environment; (c) Ask questions and ask the person to slow down or repeat the information when necessary; and (d) Paraphrase what has been said. Time is spent practicing each of these steps with conversational prompts, and homework involving real-world conversations is assigned.

Task vigilance techniques include paraphrasing and asking questions when being given instructions and using "self-talk" while working on a task. Clients are encouraged to repeat the steps of a task out loud or subvocally while performing the task in order to stay on task and remember the main steps of the task. Clients practice the self-talk technique while performing various tasks and are given homework assignments to practice these strategies while working on their own tasks at home.

## LEARNING AND MEMORY

The learning and memory sessions focus mainly on improving encoding of novel information, with a special emphasis on remembering names. The strategies taught either reduce the amount of information to be learned or make the information to be learned more meaningful. One of the primary encoding strategies is note-taking, which reduces the amount of information to be learned. For example, making a written shopping list and taking it to the store is a far more efficient use of brain resources than devoting time to memorizing a list of items to buy. The length and detail of clients' notes are reviewed to determine whether they need to write down more information or can reduce the amount of notes written.

Other encoding techniques include strategies to make new information more meaningful (e.g., paraphrasing, association of novel information with previously learned information, rhymes, visual imagery) and strategies to reduce the amount of information to be learned (e.g., chunking, categorizing, acronyms). Clients learn that there are multiple strategies for encoding all types of information and that note-taking is almost always a good option. Retrieval strategies are also reviewed, including relaxation, mental retracing, alphabetic

**FOUR PRINCIPLES:**

1) **Listen** Actively

2) **Eliminate** Distractions        "LEAP into conversations"

3) **Ask** Questions

4) **Paraphrase**

**Listen actively**

- Use nonverbal behaviors to convey that you're listening.
  - o Turn toward the speaker.
  - o Open your posture, relax, avoid "closed" body language.
  - o Lean toward the speaker.
  - o Maintain adequate eye contact.

**Eliminate distractions**

- What sorts of distractions affect your conversations? Phones? Kids? TV? Pets? How can you reduce these distractions?

**Ask questions**

- Ask questions for clarification.
- Ask the speaker to slow down, repeat information, or explain something in a different way.

**Paraphrase.**

- Repeat information back in your own words, which will help you understand, pay attention to, and remember the information later.
- Helps ensure that you've heard correctly and understand; gives the speaker a chance to correct any misunderstandings.

**Figure 9.1** Conversational attention strategies in Compensatory Cognitive Training

searching, and recreating the context in which the learning occurred. Finally, there is a section on name-learning strategies (Box 9.1) that is typically popular with clients.

## EXECUTIVE FUNCTIONING

The remaining sessions target executive functioning, focusing particularly on problem solving, cognitive flexibility, self-monitoring, and planning to meet goals and deadlines. A six-step problem-solving method is taught (Form 9.3), and detailed, personalized coaching on brainstorming is provided. Clients practice brainstorming by generating fifteen to twenty solutions to sample situations (e.g., all the ways to get a cat out of a tree), then practice brainstorming solutions to real-world problems (e.g., all the ways to look for a job; all the ways to learn the local bus routes; all the ways to save money). When clients feel confident about brainstorming, they are asked to use the six-step problem-solving method to find

Box 9.1

### Name-Learning Strategies in Compensatory Cognitive Training

A specific kind of encoding that many people have difficulty with is learning and remembering people's names. Let's talk about some strategies to help with this.

BEFORE you meet new people, mentally PREPARE yourself to remember their names by reviewing your strategies. WHEN you meet new people, do the following:

1. **OBSERVE THEM:**
   - Look people in the eye when you meet them.
   - Notice their physical characteristics; look for cues/links to their names.
2. **LISTEN** to the actual sound of the person's name when you hear it.
3. **REQUEST REPETITION** of the person's name if it is noisy or the name is unusual.
   - "I'm sorry, it's so loud in here—would you mind repeating your name?" "Could you say your name again? I've never heard it before."
   - This way you hear the name again (even if you heard it the first time!).
4. **VERIFY PRONUNCIATION** if it's noisy or the name is unusual.
   - Let me see if I'm saying that right. Is it _____?
5. **REQUEST SPELLING** (you can also do this with common names that often have multiple spellings, such as Terri, Terrie, Terry, and Teri).
   - Visualize the spelling in your head; imagine the name written down.
6. **REQUEST DERIVATION** of the name by asking suitable questions:
   - About the name's nationality ("What kind of name is Anu?").
   - About the person's preference for a nickname ("Is Bob short for Robert? Do you prefer Bob or Robert?").
   - About the history or story behind the name if it's unusual. ("It sounds like there's a story behind the name 'Brick.'").
7. **REPEAT THE NAME** in the initial conversation, either by asking questions about the name or by using the name in questions, such as, "What do you do for a living, Richard?" or "Do you have any children, Robin?"
8. **REPEAT THE NAME** when saying goodbye ("Nice to have met you, Sam.").
9. **REHEARSE** the name and **QUIZ** yourself.
10. **USE ASSOCIATION** to think about similarities and differences between the new person and other people you know who have the same name.
11. **USE IMAGERY:**
    - Sandy Brown has light brown (sandy-colored) hair.
    - Dr. Burns is bald, as if his hair burned off.
12. **USE RHYMES (and Imagery).**
    - Sandy Brown wears a frown. (Picture her frowning.)
    - Bobby Knight starts a fight. (Picture him throwing a punch.)
    - Dr. Burns always learns. (Picture him in the library with lots of books.)
13. **WRITE DOWN** names of new people (such as in a spiral notebook you carry with you).
14. **REINTRODUCE YOURSELF** to the person, and they'll introduce themselves back to you!

solutions to their own problems. Clients are asked to identify at least one problem they would like to solve, and the six-step problem-solving method is used in class and at home to address their problems or goals (e.g., How can I increase my income? How can I meet new friends?).

Cognitive flexibility is also practiced. Clients are encouraged to monitor their progress while solving problems and to change behavior accordingly through games such as "20 Questions" and sorting decks of playing cards; they then plan how to apply these skills in their own lives. Other strategies taught include self-talk while problem solving, hypothesis testing (looking for confirming and disconfirming evidence), and self-monitoring (continuing to use strategies that are working and switching strategies that are not working). Finally, clients are taught how to plan to meet goals and deadlines by working backward from the end goal or deadline, determining the steps needed to meet the goal or deadline, and assigning deadlines for these steps in their calendars (Form 9.4).

## RESULTS FROM STUDIES OF COMPENSATORY COGNITIVE TRAINING

CCT studies have now been completed in multiple populations, including people with schizophrenia (Twamley et al., 2011, 2012; Mendella et al., 2015), http://www. ncbi.nlm.nih.gov/pubmed/25631454, mood disorders (Twamley et al., 2013), hoarding disorder (Ayers et al., 2014), and traumatic brain injury (Twamley et al., 2014a, 2014b). Results thus far indicate that participating in CCT is associated with improvements in aspects of cognition, psychiatric symptoms, functional capacity, and quality of life.

In a randomized controlled trial of sixty-nine outpatients with schizophrenia who were randomly assigned to receive group-based CCT or standard pharmacotherapy, those who received CCT showed differential improvement in objectively measured attention, verbal memory, everyday functioning skills, and negative symptom severity, as well as subjective quality of life (Twamley et al., 2012). In a randomized controlled trial of 153 unemployed, work-seeking outpatients with schizophrenia ($n = 58$), bipolar disorder ($n = 37$), or major depression ($n = 58$), those who received individual CCT treatment from their employment specialist showed improvements in learning, financial capacity, depressive symptom severity, and self-reported everyday functioning (Twamley et al., 2013). Those with schizophrenia showed CCT-associated improvements in working memory and everyday functioning skills, and those with bipolar disorder showed CCT-associated improvements in psychiatric symptom severity and quality of life (Twamley et al., 2013). When paired with exposure therapy in older adults with hoarding disorder, CCT strategies doubled the response rates relative to a previous trial of cognitive behavioral therapy alone (Ayers et al., 2013). The same group-based CCT strategies, when tested in a randomized controlled trial in veterans

## 6-Step Problem-Solving Worksheet

1. Define the problem:

_____

2. Brainstorm solutions (below).
3. Evaluate the solutions.

| Solutions | Easy? | Cost OK? | Likely to work? | Other notes |
|---|---|---|---|---|
|  |  |  |  |  |
|  |  |  |  |  |
|  |  |  |  |  |
|  |  |  |  |  |
|  |  |  |  |  |
|  |  |  |  |  |
|  |  |  |  |  |
|  |  |  |  |  |
|  |  |  |  |  |
|  |  |  |  |  |
|  |  |  |  |  |
|  |  |  |  |  |
|  |  |  |  |  |
|  |  |  |  |  |
|  |  |  |  |  |

4. Select a solution (or more than one solution) to try.
5. Try out the solution(s).
6. Evaluate again. Is your problem solved? If not, try a new solution or solutions.

Example: The rent is due today and I am $20 short.

1. **Define the problem:** *Need $20 more to pay rent.*

2. **Brainstorm solutions:**
   a. *Ask landlord for an extension.*
   b. *Ask my boss for an extra shift and a cash advance of $20.*
   c. *Tell landlord I will have to move because I can't afford the rent.*
   d. *Ask landlord if I can pay $20 less this month in exchange for doing some repairs to the apartment.*
   e. *Say nothing and wait until I have the $20 to pay the rent.*

3. **Evaluate the solutions**
   a. *The landlord hasn't agreed to that in the past—unlikely to work.*
   b. *Possible—they've been needing extra help at work.*
   c. *Not really a good option—moving is expensive, and other apartments cost as much as mine.*
   d. *Possible—there is some stucco on the apartment building that needs patching.*
   e. *Not a good idea—the landlord could evict me if I don't pay the rent on time.*

4. **Select a solution to try:** *I decide to try Solution "d."*

5. **Try the solution:** *I call the landlord and explain the situation, offering to repair the stucco.*

6. **Evaluate the outcome of the solution:** *The landlord declined my offer to repair the stucco*

Back to Step 4!

4. **Select a new solution, because my first one didn't work:** *I decide to try Solution "b."*

5. **Try the solution:** *I ask my boss for an extra shift and $20 cash in advance of my paycheck.*

6. **Evaluate the outcome of the solution:** *My boss gave me an extra shift and $20 in cash. I can pay my rent on time now. My solution worked and my problem is solved.*

**Define the goal or project:**

**Example Goal:** By December 10, I will have all of my holiday cards mailed out.

_____

_____

_____

| Target Date | Step |
|---|---|
| 11/1 | Make a list of card recipients and addresses. |
| 11/5 | Purchase holiday cards. |
| 11/10 | Start writing cards, 30 minutes per night. |
| 11/20 | Have 50% of cards written. |
| 11/25 | Obtain any missing addresses. |
| 12/1 | Have all cards written and addressed. |
| 12/5 | Purchase stamps. |
| 12/10 | Mail cards. |
| | |
| | |
| | |
| | |
| | |
| | |
| | |
| | |
| | |
| | |

with traumatic brain injuries, showed positive differential effects on postconcussive symptom severity, prospective memory performance, and subjective quality of life (Twamley et al., 2014a, 2014b).

It is clinically useful to know who is likely to respond well to an intervention such as CCT. One study found that CCT-associated improvement was correlated with worse baseline scores on measures of cognitive performance, symptom severity, functional capacity, self-rated quality of life, cognitive problems, and strategy use (Twamley et al., 2011). Participants with lower baseline functioning may have more room to improve. Age has also been examined as a predictor of outcomes because of concern that older people may not improve much after cognitive training. The opposite pattern was found: Although most of the correlations between age and amount of improvement after CCT were not statistically significant, they were almost all positive, suggesting that many types of individuals can improve with CCT treatment, including older people (Twamley et al., 2011).

The following quotations from participants highlight the utility of CCT in applying new cognitive strategies to their own lives:

- *"My calendar helps me to mark off my morning pills—I can check to see that I took them."*
- *"[The calendar] gives me peace of mind. I make notes to myself about ordering prescriptions and household duties."*
- *"I went from not checking my sugars daily (maybe every other day, or I would skip a few days) to checking every day or twice a day. I write my sugar levels down in my calendar."* [From an individual with type 2 diabetes]
- *"Paraphrasing makes my conversations more interesting. Normally I would just say, 'Is that right?' but now I'm a more active participant."*
- *"I love the overlearning strategy to remember names. I made flashcards for each new person I met at my AA meetings. On the back of the card, I'll write down their phone number and personal details. . . . I'm having a social life outside of my addiction for the first time in two and a half years."*
- *"Self-talk is a learning tool. It's not like talking back to voices. If you do it for instructions or a task, it's normal."*

Two recent meta-analyses suggested that cognitive training or cognitive remediation is most effective when it is provided in the context of a broader psychosocial rehabilitation program (McGurk et al., 2007; Wykes et al., 2011). My research group has used CCT in conjunction with supported employment and supported education, and we are currently testing a combination of CCT and Cognitive Behavioral Social Skills Training (Granholm et al., 2014) to target negative symptoms and functioning. We are also testing CCT as an early intervention for youth who are at high risk for psychosis, given that younger people may be especially receptive to developing new cognitive habits.

Whether CCT is used as a stand-alone intervention or as a part of other rehabilitative services, the hope is that cognitive strategies will develop into long-term habits that generalize beyond the classroom and ultimately enhance community integration and quality of life for individuals with psychiatric illness or other cognitive impairments.

## REFERENCES

Ayers, C. R., Saxena, S., Espejo, E., Twamley, E. W., Granholm, E., Liu, L., & Wetherell, J. L. (2014). Novel treatment for geriatric hoarding disorder: An open trial of cognitive rehabilitation paired with behavior therapy. *American Journal of Geriatric Psychiatry*, *22*, 248–252.

Bayley, P. J., Frascino, J. C., & Squire, L. R. (2005). Robust habit learning in the absence of awareness and independent of the medial temporal lobe. *Nature*, *436*, 550–553.

Bellack, A. S., Mueser, K. T., Gingerich, S., & Agresta, J. (1997). *Social skills training for schizophrenia*. New York: The Guilford Press.

Choi, J., & Medalia, A. (2005). Factors associated with a positive response to cognitive remediation in a community psychiatric sample. *Psychiatric Services*, *56*, 602–604.

Clare, L., McKenna, P. J., Mortimer, A. M., & Baddeley, A. D. (1993). Memory in schizophrenia: What is impaired and what is preserved? *Neuropsychologia*, *31*, 1225–1241.

Delahunty, A., & Morice, R. (1993). *A training programme for the remediation of cognitive deficits in schizophrenia*. Albury, Australia: New South Wales Department of Health.

Duckworth, A. L., Steen, T. A., & Seligman, M. E. (2005). Positive psychology in clinical practice. *Annual Review of Clinical Psychology*, *1*, 629–651.

Granholm, E., Holden, J., Link, P. C., & McQuaid, J. R. (2014). Randomized clinical trial of cognitive behavioral social skills training for schizophrenia: Improvement in functioning and experiential negative symptoms. *Journal of Consulting and Clinical Psychology*, *82*, 1173–1185.

Green, M. F. (1996). What are the functional consequences of neurocognitive deficits in schizophrenia? *American Journal of Psychiatry*, *153*, 321–330.

Green, M. F., & Nuechterlein, K. H. (1999). Should schizophrenia be treated as a neurocognitive disorder? *Schizophrenia Bulletin*, *25*, 309–319.

Heinrichs R. W., & Zakzanis, K. K. (1998). Neurocognitive deficit in schizophrenia: A quantitative review of the evidence. *Neuropsychology*, *12*, 426–445.

Keri, S., Juhasz, A., Rimanoczy, A., Szekeres, G., Kelemen, O., Cimmer, C., . . . & Janka, Z. (2005). Habit learning and the genetics of the dopamine D3 receptor: Evidence from patients with schizophrenia and healthy controls. *Behavioral Neuroscience*, *119*, 687–693.

Kidd, S. A., Herman, Y., Barbic, S., Ganguli, R., George, T. P., Hassan, S., . . . & Velligan, D. (2014). Testing a modification of cognitive adaptation training: Streamlining the model for broader implementation. *Schizophrenia Research*, *156*, 46–50.

Knowlton, B. J., Mangels, J. A., & Squire, L. R. (1996). A neostriatal habit learning system in humans. *Science*, *273*, 1399–1402.

McGurk S. R., & Mueser, K. T. (2004). Cognitive functioning, symptoms, and work in supported employment: A review and heuristic model. *Schizophrenia Research*, *70*, 147–173.

McGurk, S. R., Twamley, E. W., Sitzer, D. I., McHugo, G. J., & Mueser, K. T. (2007). A meta-analysis of cognitive remediation in schizophrenia. *American Journal of Psychiatry, 164,* 1791–1802.

Meichenbaum, D., & Cameron, R. (1973). Training schizophrenics to talk to themselves: A means of developing attentional controls. *Behavior Therapy, 4,* 515–534.

Palmer, B. W., Heaton, R. K., Gladsjo, J. A., Evans, J. D., Patterson, T. L., Golshan, S., & Jeste, D. V. (2002). Heterogeneity in functional status among older outpatients with schizophrenia: Employment history, living situation, and driving. *Schizophrenia Research, 55,* 205–215.

Medalia, A., & Revheim, N. (2002). *Dealing with cognitive dysfunction associated with psychiatric disabilities: A handbook for families and friends of individuals with psychiatric disorders.* New York: State Office of Mental Health.

Twamley, E. W., Burton, C. Z., & Vella, L. (2011). Cognitive training for psychosis: Who benefits? Who stays in treatment? *Schizophrenia Bulletin, 37,* S55-S62.

Twamley E. W., Doshi, R. R., Nayak, G. V., Palmer, B. W., Golshan, S., Heaton, R. K., . . . & Jeste, D. V. (2002). Generalized cognitive impairments, ability to perform everyday tasks, and level of independence in community living situations of older patients with psychosis. *American Journal of Psychiatry, 159,* 2013–2020.

Twamley, E. W., Jak, A. J., Delis, D. C., Bondi, M. W., & Lohr, J. B. (2014a). Cognitive Symptom Management and Rehabilitation Therapy (CogSMART) for veterans with traumatic brain injury: A pilot randomized controlled trial. *Journal of Rehabilitation Research and Development, 51,* 59–69.

Twamley, E. W., Jeste, D. V., & Bellack, A. S. (2003). A review of cognitive training in schizophrenia. *Schizophrenia Bulletin, 29,* 359–382.

Twamley, E. W., Thomas, K. R., Gregory, A. M., Jak, A. J., Bondi, M. W., Delis, D. C., & Lohr, J. B. (2014b). CogSMART compensatory cognitive training for traumatic brain injury: Effects over 1 year. *Journal of Head Trauma Rehabilitation.* [Epub ahead of print]

Twamley, E. W., Vella, L., Burton, C. Z., Heaton, R. K., & Jeste, D. V. (2012). Compensatory cognitive training for psychosis: Effects in a randomized controlled trial. *Journal of Clinical Psychiatry, 73,* 1212–1219.

Twamley, E. W., Vella, L., Burton, C. Z., Heaton, R. K., & Jeste, D. V. (2013). Compensatory cognitive training for people with severe mental illness: Effects on cognition, functional capacity, and psychiatric symptoms. *Journal of the International Neuropsychological Society, 19*(S1), 142.

Velligan, D. I., Prihoda, T. J., Ritch, J. L., Maples, N., Bow-Thomas, C. C., & Dassori, A. (2002). A randomized single-blind pilot study of compensatory strategies in schizophrenia outpatients. *Schizophrenia Bulletin, 28,* 283.

Wykes, T., Huddy, V., Cellard, C., McGurk, S. R., & Czobor, P. (2011). A meta-analysis of cognitive remediation for schizophrenia: Methodology and effect sizes. *American Journal of Psychiatry, 168,* 472–485.

Wykes, T., Reeder, C., Corner, J., Williams, C., & Everitt, B. (1999). The effects of neurocognitive remediation on executive processing in patients with schizophrenia. *Schizophrenia Bulletin, 25,* 291–307.

# 10

# Integrating Social Cognitive Training

WILLIAM P. HORAN, DAVID L. ROBERTS, AND KATHERINE HOLSHAUSEN ∎

## INTRODUCTION

Decades of research have firmly established that neurocognitive impairment is a core feature of schizophrenia that is reliably associated with poor functional outcomes. As described in earlier chapters of this book, the functional significance of these impairments has led to major efforts to intervene at the level of neurocognition as a means of improving outcomes. Despite these important developments, it is unlikely that interventions targeting only neurocognition will be sufficient. The amount of variance in outcome that is accounted for by neurocognition is typically in the range of 20% to 40%, and the impact of cognitive remediation (CR) on functioning has thus far been modest (see Chapter 1). Thus, additional factors that contribute to poor outcome need to be identified and addressed to maximize functional recovery.

In recent years, social cognition has rapidly emerged as an important research topic that holds great promise for helping us understand and treat the causes of functional disability in schizophrenia. The term *social cognition* broadly refers to the mental operations underlying social interactions, including perceiving, interpreting, and generating responses to the behaviors, emotions, and intentions of others (Fiske & Taylor, 1991; Kunda, 1999). It encompasses a diverse set of skills that are relatively distinct from neurocognition and critical for adaptively navigating the complexities of the social environment. In clinical practice, clients with schizophrenia often describe difficulties perceiving social cues and effectively relating to others, as in the following examples:

- *"If I do something wrong I can't tell if people are mad at me. I left my last job when I made a mistake because I thought all the other people working there thought I was stupid."*

- *"I don't understand when people are joking. Sometimes I laugh when I see other people laughing, but I don't really get it."*

Consistent with these clinical descriptions, rapidly growing evidence documents substantial social cognitive impairments and biases in schizophrenia. Because social interactions are a ubiquitous part of functioning across the domains of work and school, friends and family, and daily living in the community, one would expect such disturbances to have widespread effects. Consistent with this notion, social cognitive disturbances have been found to uniquely contribute to poor functional outcomes, above and beyond neurocognition, and this has inspired a new generation of social cognitive intervention studies in schizophrenia.

Although understanding of the relationship between social cognitive training and CR is currently in its infancy, social cognitive difficulties can be expected to interface with CR in several ways. For example, they may interfere with some clients' ability to benefit from CR, which often includes group-based treatment components. Social cognitive impairments also may limit generalization of gains from CR to improvements in real world functioning. Therefore, clinicians may enhance the potential benefits of CR for their clients by considering and addressing social cognitive challenges.

This chapter comprises three main sections. First, there is a brief overview of social cognition in schizophrenia and the rationale for intervening at this level to enhance functional outcomes. Second, recent efforts to enhance social cognition through psychosocial interventions are described. Third, we consider and provide illustrative examples of how clinicians may use understanding of social cognitive deficits to more effectively implement CR and how they may most efficiently integrate social cognitive training programs with CR.

## SOCIAL COGNITION IN SCHIZOPHRENIA

### Major Domains of Social Cognition

Social cognition encompasses a large set of processes that are involved in perceiving and interpreting the behaviors, emotions, and intentions of other people. It includes processing a range of social information, from how we identify an emotion on a face to how we draw inferences about another person's goals and intentions. Research in schizophrenia has focused on four main domains of social cognition.

#### EMOTION PROCESSING

The term *emotion processing* refers to emotion perception and utilization of emotional information. An influential model of emotion processing (Salovey & Sluyter, 1997) consists of four components: (a) identifying emotions (e.g., via facial affect or vocal prosody), (b) facilitating emotions (i.e., understanding how certain emotions can assist performance on different tasks), (c) understanding emotions (i.e., understanding emotional blends and transitions), and (d) managing emotions (i.e., regulation of emotional states of self and others).

## SOCIAL PERCEPTION

The term *social perception* refers to identifying and utilizing social cues to make judgments about social roles, rules, relationships, context, or the characteristics of others (e.g., trustworthiness). This domain also includes *social knowledge*, which refers to one's knowledge of norms and schemas surrounding social situations and interactions.

## MENTALIZING

The term *mentalizing* refers to the ability to make inferences about the thoughts, beliefs, and intentions of others. This process, also referred to as Theory of Mind or mental state attribution, involves considering situations from the perspectives of other people or "standing in their shoes." Mentalizing processes are required to understand nonliteral language use, such as whether others are being sarcastic or deceptive or using metaphorical and humorous language.

## SOCIAL COGNITIVE BIAS

In some situations, people do not have access to enough information to make sound judgments, and they therefore rely on guess-making strategies or heuristics (Fiske & Taylor, 2008). These strategies are often influenced by people's situational goals, mood, and other factors, leading to biased judgments (Schwarz & Clore, 2007). The term *attributional bias* refers to the causal explanations one makes for ambiguous outcomes of life events—such as when you leave a voicemail for a friend and he does not call back. Attributions can be internal (i.e., due to oneself) or external (i.e., not due to oneself), and external attributions are further classified as either personal (i.e., due to a specific person) or situational (i.e., due to chance or situational factors). There is evidence that clients with persecutory delusions show a "personalizing bias," reflecting a tendency to attribute negative outcomes to the intentions of others rather than to situational factors (Kinderman & Bentall, 1997). Clients with delusions also show a bias toward being overconfident in their judgments, both by making hasty decisions and by holding firm to decisions in the face of contradictory evidence (Moritz & Woodward, 2006).

A variety of performance-based laboratory measures have been used to assess these aspects of social cognition in schizophrenia. The magnitude of the differences between clients and controls on capacity-based social cognitive tasks is substantial. A review of 112 studies involving 3908 clients and 3570 controls reported significant between-group differences for three of the domains with large effect sizes: emotion processing (effect size, .89), social perception (1.04), and mentalizing (.96) (Savla, Vella, Armstrong, Penn, & Twamley, 2013). Although research has been conducted primarily with chronically ill clients, social cognitive impairments are also detectable in unmedicated clients and those with recent-onset schizophrenia (McCleery, Horan, & Green, 2014). Further, the differences are relatively stable across acutely symptomatic and remitted states and across phases of the illness, suggesting that social cognitive impairments are likely core features of the illness and not simply a result of medication side effects or clinical episodes.

Research on social cognitive biases has been more equivocal, with roughly the same number of studies showing differences and no differences between clients and controls (Savla et al., 2013). This finding is surprising in light of the clinical face validity of these biases in schizophrenia—they overlap considerably with the symptom constructs of paranoia and delusions. However, because biases are influenced by people's interpersonal goals, they are notoriously difficult to measure with self-report and performance-based instruments. For example, paranoid clients who are motivated to be seen as normal may appear to "fake good" on measures of social cognitive bias (Roberts, Fiszdon, DeGeorge, & Tek, 2009; Roberts & Penn, 2009).

## Relation to Functional Outcome

Because social cognition is so central to understanding and effectively interacting with other people, problems such as misperceptions and unexpected reactions to and from other people would be expected to adversely impact functioning across a variety of domains. In support of this expectation, three lines of evidence indicate that social cognitive impairments do indeed make important and unique contributions to functional outcome in schizophrenia.

### CORRELATIONS WITH FUNCTIONAL OUTCOME

Abnormal performance on social cognitive tasks is consistently related to various aspects of social competence and functioning in people with schizophrenia. A review of fifty-two studies that included 2692 people (Fett et al., 2011) documented relatively strong correlations between outcome and the social cognitive domains described earlier: emotion processing ($r = 0.31$), social perception ($r = 0.41$), and mental state attribution or Theory of Mind ($r = 0.48$). Furthermore, in studies that directly compared the explanatory value of social cognition versus neurocognition, social cognitive measures accounted for an average of 16% of the variance in community functioning, which was significantly larger than the 6% of variance accounted for by composite measures of neurocognition.

### ADDED VALUE OF SOCIAL COGNITION

Because social cognition and neurocognition are both associated with functioning, a fundamental question is whether they make separate, unique contributions to outcome. Neurocognitive and social cognitive tasks often share cognitive processes, such as working memory and perception, and therefore are clearly associated. Indeed, significant correlations are found between performance on measures of social cognition and neurocognition (Pinkham & Penn, 2006; Sergi & Green, 2002). However, the magnitude of these relations is generally moderate, and statistical models fit better when the two domains are separated than when they are combined (Bell, Tsang, Greig, & Bryson, 2009; Sergi et al., 2007). In addition to evidence that these domains are separable, social cognition shows *unique* relationships to outcome, contributing incremental variance to the prediction of real-world functioning above and beyond that provided by neurocognition (Couture, Penn, & Roberts, 2006; Mancuso, Horan, Kern, & Green, 2011; Pinkham & Penn, 2006). The conclusion that there is both partial overlap and relative distinctiveness between neurocognition and social cognition is consistent with social neuroscience research, which reveals partially overlapping and partially distinct patterns of neural activation associated with nonsocial and social cognitive activation tasks (Van Overwalle, 2009).

### Social Cognition as a Mediator

Aside from the question of whether social cognition and neurocognition uniquely contribute to functional outcome, researchers have also examined the issue of *how* they interact to impact outcome. There has until recently been a substantial gap in understanding of the mechanisms through which neurocognitive deficits measured in the laboratory ultimately give rise to the functional deficits clients experience in their daily lives in the community. Using statistical modeling approaches, researchers have tested the hypothesis that social cognition mediates the link between neurocognitive impairments on the one hand and functional outcome on the other hand. As illustrated in Figure 10.1, rather than predicting a direct causal relationship between neurocognition and outcome, this mediation model hypothesizes that neurocognition influences social cognition, which in turn influences functional outcome.

This role of social cognition as a mediator is now supported by a large number of studies. A review by Schmidt, Mueller, and Roder (2011) indicated that in 14 out of 15 studies, social cognition was a significant mediator between neurocognition and functional outcome. This demonstrates that social cognition is a key intervening mechanism through which neurocognitive deficits ultimately affect functioning. In other words, social cognition is more proximal to outcome than is neurocognition in the chain of causal factors that ultimately lead to poor functional outcome. As discussed later in this chapter, the proximity of social cognition to outcome suggests that improvements in this domain

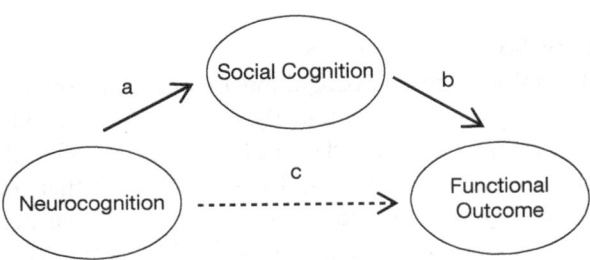

**Figure 10.1** Mediation model. The relationship between neurocognition and functional outcome is mediated by social cognition in schizophrenia.

may be particularly strong in terms of generalization to improvements in daily functioning.

In summary, there is substantial evidence that people with schizophrenia experience social cognitive disturbances, which consistently show robust and distinctive relations to functioning. Social cognition also acts as a mediator between neurocognition and outcome, indicating that it is an important intervening variable in the pathway to recovery. These findings support the value of social cognition as an important target for treatments aimed at helping clients achieve a full functional recovery.

## SOCIAL COGNITIVE TRAINING APPROACHES IN SCHIZOPHRENIA

Given the link between social cognition and functional outcome, there has been growing interest in developing psychosocial interventions to enhance social cognition in schizophrenia. This section describes the types of treatment approaches that have been developed specifically to target social cognition and then summarizes the research on the efficacy of these treatments. Many of the social cognitive interventions reviewed here incorporate training techniques that are also fundamental to CR, including shaping, scaffolding, self-instruction, positive feedback, graded increases in task difficulty, errorless learning, and teaching of information processing strategies. In addition, some social cognitive interventions use novel techniques derived from social cognitive research that have no overlap with CR techniques. Examples of the latter include mimicry of emotional expressions and emotional self-monitoring.

### Social Cognitive Intervention Techniques

Two treatment packages that exemplify the range of social cognitive intervention techniques are Social Cognitive Skills Training (SCST; Horan et al., 2011) and Social Cognition and Interaction Training (SCIT; Penn, Roberts, Combs, & Sterne, 2007). Both interventions target multiple domains of social cognition, including emotion processing, social perception, mentalizing, and social cognitive bias. Also, both use a group format (typically involving five to seven clients) that allows for discussion and debate about photographic and video stimuli, and both support the use of games and other interactive exercises to practice social cognitive skills and to apply them in a social context. The following sections describe the types of training exercises that are used within the four targeted domains of social cognition.

#### EMOTION PROCESSING

The most well-established social cognitive interventions for schizophrenia are those designed to improve face emotion perception. SCST and SCIT use a common set of techniques built on the foundation of drill-and-repeat practice, in which clients repeatedly judge the emotions shown in a series of pictured faces. In SCST, clients are taught to divide each face into three regions (forehead/eyebrows, eyes/eyelids, and nose/mouth) and then, within each region, to focus on key facial cues that characterize specific emotions (e.g., smile = happy, frown = sad). Clients practice interpreting whole faces as well as images depicting only selected regions of the face (See Figure 10.2). This gives clients practice in interpreting specific social cues rather than relying on holistic impressions that may lead to hasty judgments. As in SCST, SCIT clients learn to associate specific facial cues with basic emotions. Added to this is practice in facial mimicry, in which clients attempt to mirror others' facial expressions on their own face in order to make better judgments. This technique is thought to recruit proprioceptive feedback processes that are rooted in specialized social cognitive neurocircuitry (Penn & Combs, 2000). SCIT also uses an emotion attention shaping approach (Combs et al., 2009) in which visual prompts cue trainees to focus their gaze on the central region of the face that includes the most important social information (i.e., the brow, eyes, and mouth; See Figure 10.3).

In both SCST and SCIT, clients learn to use verbalization and self-instruction during emotion perception training. This helps to reinforce strategy use and helps clients avoid social cognitive biases, such as the tendency to assume that one's initial judgment of another person's emotion is the right answer. Over the course of training, clients are challenged to make emotion perception judgments using different sensory modalities and increasingly complex stimuli (e.g., video segments rather than static photographs) (See Figure 10.4) and to move from slow,

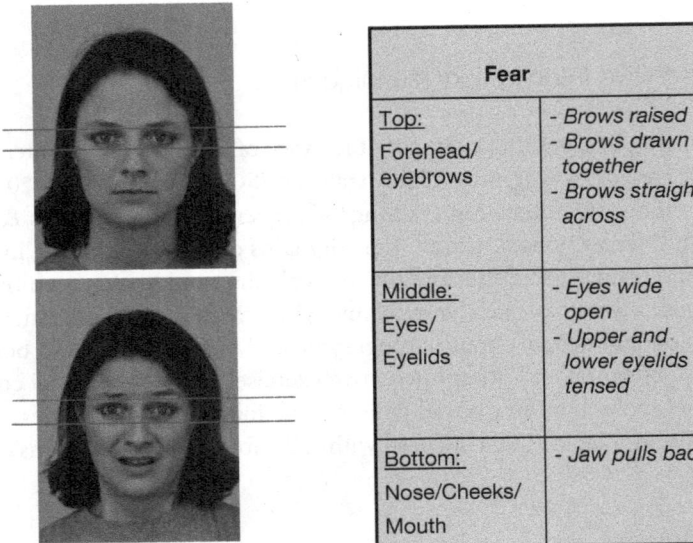

**Figure 10.2** Emotion Perception Training. Clients learn to divide faces into three regions and focus on cues within each region that are associated with specific emotions.

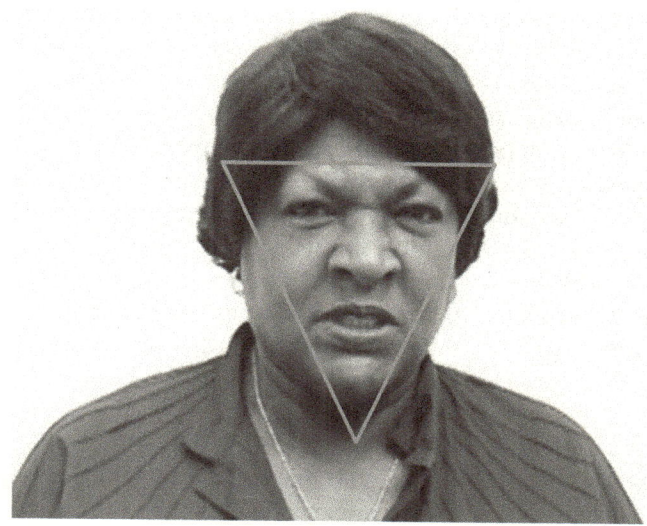

**Figure 10.3** Emotion Attention Shaping. Instructions to trainee: "Most emotions are found in the center part of the face: eyes, nose, and mouth area. Look in the upside down triangle area. Is this woman feeling happy, angry, afraid, sad, ashamed, or disgusted?"

verbally-mediated emotion *interpretation*, to faster, more fluid and automatic emotion *perception*.

### SOCIAL PERCEPTION

To address the domain of social perception, SCST and SCIT teach techniques for evaluating complex social situations using pictures, videos, and stories of people

| Emotion | Quality | Volume |
|---|---|---|
| Happy | Sing-songy and bright | Loud |
| Afraid | Jittery and breathy | Medium to soft |
| Sad | Soft & shrinking droopy | Soft |
| Angry | Bang-bang-bang | Loud |
| Disgusted | Scratchy and drawn out | Medium |
| Surprise | skyrocketing | Loud |

Practice saying
*"Did you see that?"*
with each emotion

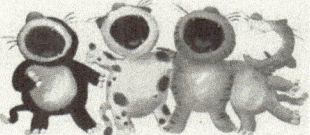

**Figure 10.4** Detecting Emotion from Vocal Quality. In SCST, clients learn vocal cues that are associated with different emotions. As with mimicry of facial emotion expressions, clients practice uttering these vocal cues to to improve their ability to recognize emotions in others and to communicate emotions to others.

interacting. A "social detective" approach is used in which clients learn to evaluate social situations like detectives attempting to solve a crime, including carefully collecting objective data (e.g., the facial cue of a frown), generating hypotheses based on data ("She is sad"), iteratively checking hypotheses against additional contextual information (e.g., "She is dressed like a clown; other people are laughing"), and updating judgments ("She is pretending to be sad"). SCST emphasizes the technique of evaluating the congruence between different pieces of information in social situations. For example, clients might notice that a woman frowning is incongruent with the fact that those around her are laughing, leading to the hypothesis that she may be feigning sadness. During this phase, SCST also teaches clients to attend to gestures and body posture to help infer others' thoughts and feelings.

## MENTALIZING

Mentalizing exercises build on the strategies discussed earlier to help clients interpret others' thoughts and intentions in increasingly complex social situations. For example, in SCST, clients practice figuring out whether others are telling white lies or being sarcastic by integrating the "5 W's" of social situations: who, what, when, where, and why. This requires clients to synthesize previously learned strategies of emotion perception and social perception. In SCIT, there is an exercise modified from the game "20 Questions" in which clients must continually update their guesses about another person's thoughts based on new answers to questions and must formulate new questions to gather evidence and test hypotheses until they have enough information to be confident in their judgments.

## SOCIAL COGNITIVE BIAS

Whereas some interventions use distinct techniques to target different social cognitive biases (e.g., attributional bias, jumping to conclusions, bias against disconfirmatory evidence; Moritz & Woodward, 2006), SCST and SCIT use the term "jumping to conclusions" as a broad label to refer to the general problem of social cognitive bias. This term is useful because clients generally know it and have a basic understanding of its meaning when they begin treatment.

In one debiasing technique, called *Separating Facts from Guesses*, the group facilitator helps clients to frame jumping to conclusions as a problem in which a person treats a guess about a social situation as if it were a fact (e.g., "I know that you don't like me"). As shown in Figure 10.5, clients practice separating social facts from guesses in pictures and videos, assigning confidence ratings to facts and guesses and learning to avoid overconfidence in unsupported guesses. Another debiasing technique is called *Generating Alternatives*. Many clients jump to conclusions because they find it difficult to imagine alternative explanations for an event. As shown in Figure 10.6, to make it easy for clients to imagine alternatives, SCIT and SCST teach clients to generate interpretations from three basic perspectives (fictional characters) that represent internal ("My-fault Mary"), external-personal ("Blaming Bill"), and external-situational ("Easy Eddie") causal attributions. Clients develop fluency in generating alternatives by applying these

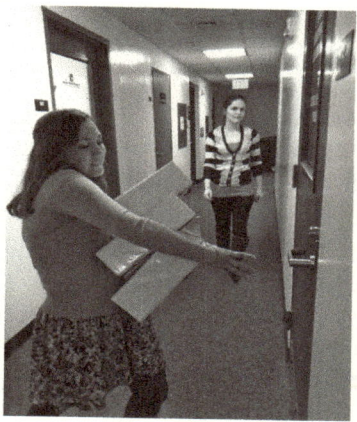

**Definitions**

Fact

- You are 100% sure it is true.
- You can see it, here it or touch it.
- Everybody in group agrees it is a fact.

Guess

- You are less than 100% sure.
- You cannot perceive it directly.
  – EG: Other's thoughts and feelings
- Guesses that are supported by several facts receive higher confidence ratings
- Some group members think it may not be true.

**Figure 10.5** Separating Facts from Guesses. Is it a fact or a guess that the woman in the foreground wants to open the door? Answer: It is a guess that the woman wants to open the door because we cannot directly perceive her wants or desires. We can only see her appearance and behavior. Based on the facts that her arm is extended and that her eyes are looking toward the door handle, we may have high confidence (e.g., 75%) in the guess that she wants to open the door. However, other guesses are also possible-such as that she just closed the door. Through repeated practice, clients learn to apply this approach to their own judgments and to catch themselves before they become overconfident about guesses that have little factual support.

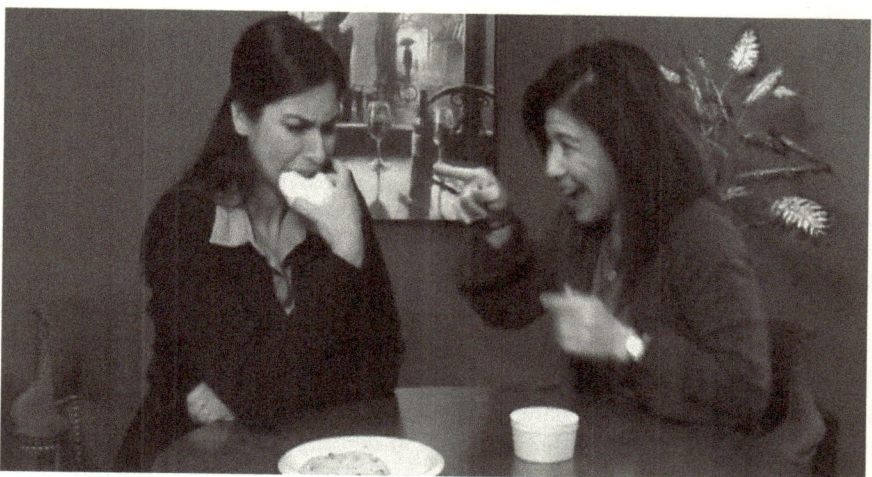

**Figure 10.6** Generating Alternatives. SCIT teaches clients to generate interpretations from three basic perspectives that represent internal, external-personal, and external-situational causal attributions: *My-fault Mary* always believes that she herself has caused an interpersonal problem and feels guilty or sad; *Blaming Bill* always believes that somebody else has caused a problem for him and he feels angry; *Easy Eddie* always believes that nobody is to blame because any problem was caused by an accident. In a typical exercise, clients would be asked to tell a story about this picture in which the woman on the left is thinking and feeling like Blaming Bill, a second story in which she is feeling like My-fault Mary, and a third in which she is feeling like Easy Eddie.

three perspectives to a series of social photographs and videos and, ultimately, to situations in their own lives.

## GENERALIZATION

Both SCST and SCIT are structured so that exercises become increasingly difficult and self-relevant over time. For example, in the final phase of SCIT, clients apply learned skills to interpret social situations in their everyday lives. This exercise serves a useful bridging function, but it also presents its own important challenges because clients are more likely to experience strong emotions and maladaptive social cognitive biases when examining their own personal experiences. For example, if a client were reprimanded by her supervisor at work, she would be likely to feel shame (or anger) about the situation. This emotion may lead her to have an exaggerated view of her own incompetence (or her supervisor's cruelty). To help with generalization, SCST and SCIT use out-of-group work and booster sessions. For example, in SCIT, clients work with a "practice partner," an acquaintance or relative who helps the client apply skills in the home environment. Along these lines, ongoing studies of SCST are testing whether the addition of "in vivo" training sessions that are conducted in the community outside the clinic (e.g., coffee shops, shopping mall) can enhance generalization of treatment benefits.

## Research Findings

Although social cognitive intervention for schizophrenia is a new area, early research on its effects has been promising. A meta-analysis of nineteen controlled treatment trials (Kurtz & Richardson, 2012) found that interventions yielded moderate to large effects on functional outcome ($d = 0.78$). This effect size surpasses average effects of CR trials on functional outcome, and social cognitive training appears to have a particular advantage over CR in effects on social functioning (compared with instrumental and vocational domains). Thus, social cognitive training may be a particularly promising adjunct to CR among individuals for whom improved interpersonal functioning is a primary treatment goal.

Regarding social cognitive domains, interventions have produced large effects on face emotion perception ($d = 0.71$ to $1.01$) and small to moderate effects on mentalizing ($d = 0.46$). Effects have thus far been minimal for attributional bias and social perception. This pattern of results supports the efficacy of the established learning approaches that are used in emotion perception training, such as drill-and-repeat practice and errorless learning. It also reflects the more concrete and "face valid" nature of emotion perception strategies. That is, in emotion perception training, clients typically are taught to apply a finite set of black-and-white rules (e.g., smile = happy, frown = sad) to consistent stimuli (pictures of faces), and they must select from a narrow set of possible responses (happy, angry, sad, surprised, afraid). It is more challenging to use simple rules of this sort to address the more complex and less tangible domains of social perception, mentalizing, and attributional bias.

The relatively weaker effects in these latter domains may also reflect measurement problems. Many interventions for these domains are intended to help clients to gather and flexibly evaluate social information but not necessarily to generate correct answers. However, most treatment trials have only measured changes in accuracy. Limitations in social cognitive assessment are a well-known issue, and refinements are in the works (Pinkham et al., 2014).

In summary, social cognitive interventions have been developed to target the full range of social cognitive abnormalities in schizophrenia. As illustrated by SCST and SCIT, interventions are designed not only to help clients make more accurate social judgments but also to help them think in a more flexible, self-aware manner while making social judgments. Although this is a young field, research on the effectiveness of social cognitive interventions has been promising, especially in the areas of functional outcome and emotion perception. In the next section, we discuss how social cognitive training approaches may interact with CR.

## INTERFACE BETWEEN SOCIAL COGNITION AND COGNITIVE REMEDIATION

The degree to which social cognition plays a role in CR is in large part determined by the specific type of CR under consideration. On the one hand, some of the pioneering treatments that addressed social cognition, such as Interpersonal Therapy (IPT; Roder, Mueller, Spaulding, & Brenner, 2010) and Cognitive Enhancement Therapy (CET; Hogarty & Flesher, 1999), included modules specifically designed to target social cognition in conjunction with neurocognition. On the other hand, some CR interventions (e.g., several early CR approaches and neuroplasticity-targeted interventions) focus exclusively on "cold" cognitive training; social cognition is not considered and has little apparent relevance to the primary goals of treatment. In line with growing evidence that social cognition is an integral part of adaptive community functioning, CR programs are increasingly incorporating social cognitive training exercises (Cognitive Remediation Experts Workshop, Florence, Italy, April, 2010). This fusion of CR and social cognitive training demonstrates a clear movement in the CR field toward enhancing generalization of cognitive abilities across a broader array of real-world settings.

Social cognitive skill deficits and biases may interface with CR in at least two ways. First, social cognitive disturbances can be an impediment to treatment delivery by diminishing clients' ability to engage in and benefit from CR training activities. Second, social cognitive disturbances may serve as a rate-limiting factor for the generalization of any cognitive gains acquired through CR to improvements in real-world functioning. In the following sections, we consider examples of how social cognitive difficulties can play out when one is working with clients in CR programs, discuss social cognitive impairments as a rate-limiting factor for generalization, and review approaches to combining social cognition training with CR.

## Social Cognition Deficits as an Impediment to Implementing Cognitive Remediation

Social cognitive difficulties manifest in various ways during social interactions, including difficulties perceiving others' facial affect and vocal tone, misunderstanding of and failure to consider the point of view of others, and biases in the interpretation of social events. In the context of CR, these types of difficulties may come up during one-on-one interactions with a therapist or during group-based activities included in some CR programs. For example, a client who is explaining the strategies that were used during a given CR task may interpret a therapist's neutral expression as angry or disappointed. This may make the client less likely to openly discuss strategies and approaches in CR exercises.

Likewise, a client could misinterpret a joke that involves metaphorical or sarcastic language. After an exercise that is completed quickly with full success, a therapist might say with the intent of sarcasm: "Well, it looks like you had a really hard time with that!" Although the therapist may intend to provide praise and reinforcement, a client could interpret this statement literally and conclude that the therapist is being critical. These types of misunderstandings can disrupt the therapeutic alliance and detract from the client's engagement, thereby impeding the client's ability to gain from CR. For these reasons, it is very useful for CR therapists to be aware of the types of social cognitive difficulties that clients with schizophrenia commonly experience and to take steps to avoid or repair any miscommunications that result from them.

Another area where social cognitive difficulties can impact CR involves bridging groups (see Chapter 4). Bridging groups typically involve efforts to apply newly developed cognitive skills to personally relevant real-world situations (e.g., using problem solving and sequencing skills to shop for groceries or prepare a meal). Although conducting these activities in a group format can be an extremely useful way for group members to benefit from shared experiences, social cognitive difficulties may be particularly likely to arise in this type of situation. Misperceptions or inaccurate attributions for other group members' behaviors can be distracting and stressful, detracting from participants' ability to attend to and fully benefit from training exercises. Consider the scenario depicted in Figure 10.7. In a group setting, one client may notice that another group member looks angry. Through a faulty attribution, she may mistakenly perceive that the group member is mad at her. This may make her feel uncomfortable, and she may withdraw from contributing to group activities and discussions. The misperception of anger toward oneself could hamper engagement in a group setting, thereby affecting group morale and individual progress.

As another example, one client may be overzealous to share in a group context, contributing more than others to the point that he becomes disruptive and prevents others from contributing to group discussions. He may not notice the annoyed looks on others' faces and may fail to consider others' perspective that it is frustrating when he talks all the time. This behavior may negatively affect the group dynamic and how often group members are willing and able to contribute

**Social Stimulus**

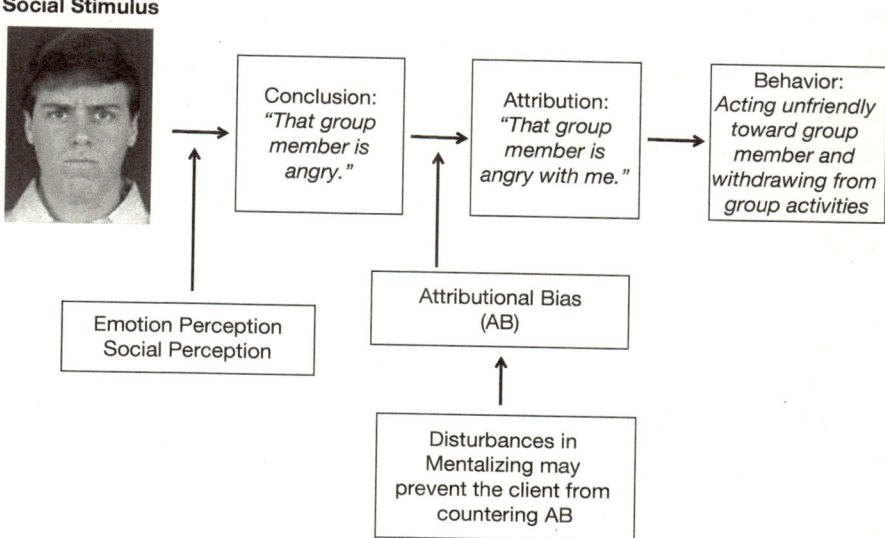

Figure 10.7 Illustration of the Conceptual Framework for the Link Between Social Cognition and Social Functioning in a Group Setting

to group discussions. It is important for the therapist to recognize that this type of behavior may be related to social cognitive deficits and be sensitive to how this issue is broached to ensure that the client understands others' perspectives.

Social cognitive difficulties can clearly create a number of challenges for optimal delivery of individual or group-based CR exercises. Although these types of difficulties are familiar to many therapists working in the field, techniques for effectively addressing them are only starting to become a formalized aspect of CR. Importantly, the potential benefit of formally addressing social cognition is likely to go far beyond facilitating optimal delivery of existing CR exercises. As described in the next section, incorporating social cognitive intervention approaches may be necessary for the benefits of CR to meaningfully generalize to improved daily functioning in the community.

## Social Cognition as a Rate-Limiting Factor for Generalization

As detailed in Chapter 1, CR programs show promising effects on measures of neurocognition, but the extent to which these gains generalize to improvements in real-world functioning has thus far been modest. As described earlier in this chapter, substantial evidence now indicates that social cognition mediates the relationship between neurocognition and functional outcome. Conceptually, this means that social cognition is one critically important mechanism through which neurocognitive abilities ultimately affect adaptive functioning in daily life. This intuitively makes sense when one considers how central social interactions are for functioning across the domains of work and school, family and friends, and daily independent living (e.g., shopping, using public transportation, living with others).

The mediating role of social cognition also has an important practical implication for CR. Specifically, the presence of social cognitive skills is critical for neurocognitive abilities to have an impact on functioning. If social cognition is not addressed, the potential benefits of any neurocognitive gains for real-world functioning may not be fully realized. To illustrate this point, consider two examples.

1. Some clients are strong in terms of nonsocial cognitive abilities required to perform tasks but are unable to obtain or keep a job due to social difficulties at work: *George has been working on cognitive flexibility in CR. He uses flexibility in the development of strategies to navigate CR computer-based exercises and also to apply these strategies in his everyday life. Increased flexibility in his approach to tasks means that George should be better able to think of multiple strategies to solve problems when they come up in the real world. A possible challenge related to social cognitive dysfunction is that George still has attributional bias and a tendency to jump to conclusions. This may lead to continued cognitive inflexibility in interpersonal contexts despite improved flexibility in neurocognitive training. For example, George may persist in using an inefficient strategy at work after his boss has shown him a better approach—not because he lacks the neurocognitive flexibility to switch his routine, but because he misinterprets his boss' suggestion as an effort to undermine him.*

2. Some clients have the desire for friends and the ability to make plans with friends in their free time but have difficulties connecting and maintaining relationships: *Before CR, Rachel was unable to go to community events because she became overwhelmed by the difficulty of planning bus routes and remembering to get off at the right stop. Now, Rachel has strategies that help her to plan trips and remember the right bus stops, but she doesn't know how to initiate conversations with people or maintain a relationship once it starts. Rachel finds herself struggling to know when it's her turn to talk in a conversation or what she should say to someone because she isn't sure how that person is feeling.*

As these vignettes illustrate, the social cognitive skills required to navigate most work and recreational activities fall outside of the purview of conventional CR approaches. For George and Rachel, developing neurocognitive skills will not be sufficient for achieving their personal goals. Instead, it will be necessary to equip them with the social cognitive skills necessary to use their enhanced neurocognitive skills in real-world settings. But how should CR and social cognitive training be integrated to maximize community functioning? We consider this issue in the final section.

## Combining Cognitive Remediation and Social Cognition Training

It is currently an open question as to how CR and social cognition training should be optimally combined, and many configurations are possible. For example, the two types of training could be provided either simultaneously or sequentially. The format of social cognitive training can vary, ranging from group-based interventions to individual training through computerized exercises. In addition, the specific domain or domains of social cognition that are addressed can vary. Currently, the data for evaluating the various possible configurations are very limited.

The feasibility of combining CR and social cognitive training has actually been documented for more than 2 decades. Some of the earliest efforts to train social cognition, including IPT and CET, used a hierarchical approach in which social cognitive training was incorporated atop neurocognitive training in the context of relatively lengthy (i.e., at least 12 months) participation in multifaceted treatment programs. In IPT, this was achieved by first targeting basic cognitive skills (e.g., attention, memory, cognitive flexibility), which were then used as a foundation to work on skills such as emotion and social perception. The relations between these two sets of thinking skills were discussed and put into action through role-playing and group-based exercises. Similarly, CET capitalized on initial basic neurocognitive skill acquisition by using those gains as a scaffolding on which more complex social cognitive skill development was superimposed. CET promoted the use of several social cognitive skills, including "gistful thinking" (i.e., understanding the themes and meanings of social messages) and motivational accounts of behavior (i.e., giving a clear account of the intentions underlying one's own and others' actions), through group-based exercises and social problem solving in real-life situations. It is noteworthy that both IPT and CET employed approaches similar to bridging to support the generalization of skills to real-life situations. As previously noted, IPT and CET are relatively lengthy, resource-intensive treatments; they are costly and require strong commitments from both patients and treatment providers, which may affect their utility in modern health care systems.

More recently, proof-of-principle studies of novel combinations of social cognitive and neurocognitive interventions have demonstrated the beneficial additive effect of computerized social cognitive training exercises. Lindenmayer et al. (2013) randomized clients into CR alone or CR plus social cognition training, using a well established but older CR program (i.e., COGPACK; Marker, 1996) and a computerized emotion perception intervention. Clients in the combined intervention achieved significant gains in both neurocognition and social cognition, demonstrating the additive effects of treating both domains. In a study with a more contemporary CR computer program, Sacks et al. (2013) similarly found that clients who engaged in an auditory-based CR program plus computerized social cognition training (i.e., facial emotion identification, social discrimination, simple social perception, and mentalizing tasks) made gains in both neurocognitive and social cognitive domains. These improvements were also related to increased neural activity in relevant regions (e.g., amygdala, postcentral gyrus) during an emotion recognition task administered before and after treatment (Hooker et al., 2012, 2013).

Looking forward, some researchers are developing and testing social cognitive training programs that capitalize on established CR training approaches. For example, Nahum et al. (2014) reported promising initial findings for a computerized training program that aims to improve affect perception, social cue perception, mentalizing, and self-referential processing using the principles of neuroplasticity-based learning. In research spearheaded by Joanna Fiszdon, the potential benefit of applying learning principles from CR, including errorless learning and scaffolding, to purely social cognitive content is being evaluated. We expect that research in this area will expand considerably in the next few years. As the field progresses, it will also be useful to incorporate individualized assessments of clients' neurocognitive and social cognitive strengths and weaknesses and personal life goals when developing treatment plans, because a single approach is unlikely to optimally fit all.

## CONCLUSIONS AND FUTURE DIRECTIONS

Understanding of the functional significance of social cognitive impairments in schizophrenia has grown dramatically over the past decade. It is now widely recognized that social cognitive impairments play a unique role in the pathways that lead to poor functioning and represent an important target for intervention. There have already been a number of promising initial efforts to address these impairments through various psychosocial treatment approaches. Findings are particularly strong for less complex social cognitive skills such as facial emotion perception. Further development of exercises to address higher-level social cognitive domains is needed. Several of the intervention strategies may be useful for clinicians to consider and apply to enhance the effectiveness of delivering CR to clients.

Further consideration of the potential synergy between social cognitive and neurocognitive treatments is a topic that is rich for development. Social cognitive impairments can affect the implementation and generalization of CR in a variety of ways. Integrating social cognitive and CR approaches therefore seems to be a highly promising approach. Systematic research is needed to identify the optimal configuration to implement these approaches in combination or to identify individual client characteristics that could be matched to particular configurations. Continued treatment development in the area of social cognition and its integration with CR approaches shows great promise for helping clients achieve a more complete functional recovery.

## REFERENCES

Bell, M., Tsang, H. W., Greig, T. C., & Bryson, G. J. (2009). Neurocognition, social cognition, perceived social discomfort, and vocational outcomes in schizophrenia. *Schizophrenia Bulletin, 35*(4), 738–747.

Cognitive Remediation Experts Workshop. (2010, April).

Combs, D. R., Tosheva, A., Penn, D. L., Basso, M. R., Wanner, J. L., & Laib, K. (2009). Attention-shaping as a means to improve emotion perception deficits in schizophrenia. *Schizophrenia Research, 105*(1–3), 68–77.

Couture, S. M., Penn, D. L., & Roberts, D. L. (2006). The functional significance of social cognition in schizophrenia: A review. *Schizophrenia Bulletin, 32*(suppl. 1), s44–s63.

Fett, A. K., Viechtbauer, W., Dominguez, M. D., Penn, D. L., van Os, J., & Krabbendam, L. (2011). The relationship between neurocognition and social cognition with functional outcomes in schizophrenia: A meta-analysis. *Neuroscience and Biobehavioral Reviews, 35*, 573–588.

Fiske, S. T., & Taylor, S. E. (1991). *Social cognition* (2nd ed.). New York: McGraw-Hill.

Fiske, S. T., & Taylor S. E. (2008). *Social cognition: From brains to culture.* Thousand Oaks, CA: Sage Publications.

Hogarty, G. E., & Flesher, S. (1999). Practice principles of cognitive enhancement therapy for schizophrenia. *Schizophrenia Bulletin, 25*(4), 693–708.

Hooker, C. I., Bruce, L., Fisher, M., Verosky, S. C., Miyakawa, A., D'esposito, M., & Vinogradov, S. (2013). The influence of combined cognitive plus social-cognitive training on amygdala response during face emotion recognition in schizophrenia. *Psychiatry Research: Neuroimaging, 213*(2), 99–107.

Hooker, C. I., Bruce, L., Fisher, M., Verosky, S. C., Miyakawa, A., & Vinogradov, S. (2012). Neural activity during emotion recognition after combined cognitive plus social cognitive training in schizophrenia. *Schizophrenia Research, 139*(1), 53–59.

Horan, W. P., Kern, R. S., Tripp, C., Hellemann, G., Wynn, J. K., Bell, M., . . . & Green, M. F. (2011). Efficacy and specificity of social cognitive skills training for outpatients with psychotic disorders. *Journal of Psychiatric Research, 45*(8), 1113–1122.

Kinderman, P., & Bentall, R. P. (1997). Causal attributions in paranoia and depression: Internal, personal, and situational attributions for negative events. *Journal of Abnormal Psychology, 106*(2), 341–345.

Kunda, Z. (1999). *Social cognition: Making sense of people.* Cambridge, MA: MIT Press.

Kurtz M. M., & Richardson, C. L. (2012). Social cognitive training for schizophrenia: A meta-analytic investigation of controlled research. *Schizophrenia Bulletin, 38*(5), 1092–1094.

Lindenmayer, J. P., McGurk, S. R., Khan, A., Kkaushik, S., Thanju, A., Hoffman, L., . . . & Hermann, E. (2013). Improving social cognition in schizophrenia: A pilot intervention combining social cognition training with cognitive remediation. *Schizophrenia Bulletin, 39*(3), 507–517.

Mancuso, F., Horan, W. P., Kern, R. S., & Green, M. F. (2011). Social cognition in psychosis: Multidimensional structure, clinical correlates, and relationship with functional outcome. *Schizophrenia Research, 125*, 143–151.

Marker, K. R. (1996). *COGPACK: Programmpaket für Neuropsychologischen Rehabilitation.* Ladenburg, Germany: Marker Software.

McCleery, A., Horan, W. P., & Green, M. F. (2014). Social cognition in early phase schizophrenia. In P. Lysaker, G. Dimaggio, & M. Brüne (Eds.), *Social cognition and metacognition in schizophrenia: Psychopathology and treatment approaches* (pp. 50–63). Amsterdam: Elsevier.

Moritz, S., & Woodward, T. S. (2006). A generalized bias against disconfirmatory evidence in schizophrenia. *Psychiatry Research, 142*(2–3), 157–165.

Nahum, M., Fisher, M., Loewy, R., Poelke, G., Ventura, J., Nuechterlein, K. H., . . . & Vinogradov, S. (2014). A novel, online social cognitive training program for young adults with schizophrenia: A pilot study. *Schizophrenia Research: Cognition, 1*(1), e11–e19. doi:10.1016/j.scog.2014.01.003

Penn, D. L., & Combs, D. (2000). Modification of affect perception deficits in schizophrenia. *Schizophrenia Research, 46*(2–3), 217–229.

Penn, D. L., Roberts, D. L., Combs, D., & Sterne, A. (2007). Best practices: The development of the Social Cognition and Interaction Training (SCIT) program for schizophrenia-spectrum disorders. *Psychiatric Services, 58*(4), 449–452.

Pinkham, A. E., & Penn, D. L. (2006). Neurocognitive and social cognitive predictors of interpersonal skill in schizophrenia. *Psychiatry Research, 143,* 167–178.

Pinkham, A. E., Penn, D. L., Green, M. F., Buck, B., Healey, K., & Harvey, P. D. (2014). The social cognition psychometric evaluation study: Results of the expert survey and RAND panel. *Schizophrenia Bulletin, 40*(4), 813–823.

Roberts, D. L., Fiszdon, J. M., DeGeorge, P., & Tek, C. (2009). Impression-management effects in paranoia assessment. *Schizophrenia Bulletin, 35*(suppl. 1), s2–s3.

Roberts, D. L. & Penn, D. L. (2009). Social Cognition and Interaction Training (SCIT) for outpatients with schizophrenia: A preliminary study. *Psychiatry Research, 166*(2–3), 141–147.

Roder, V., Mueller, D. R., Spaulding, W., & Brenner, H. D. (2010). *Integrated psychological therapy (IPT) for schizophrenia clients* (2nd ed.). Goettingen/Cambridge, MA: Hogrefe.

Sacks, S., Fisher, M., Garrett, C., Alexander, P., Holland, C., Rose, D., . . . & Vinogradov, S. (2013). Combining computerized social cognitive training with neuroplasticity-based auditory training in schizophrenia. *Clinical Schizophrenia and Related Psychoses, 7*(2), 78–86A.

Salovey, P., & Sluyter, D. J. (1997). *Emotional development and emotional intelligence.* New York: Basic Books.

Savla, G. N., Vella, L., Armstrong, C. C., Penn, D. L., & Twamley, E. W. (2013). Deficits in domains of social cognition in schizophrenia: A meta-analysis of the empirical literature. *Schizophrenia Bulletin, 39,* 979–992.

Schmidt, S. J., Mueller, D. R., & Roder, V. (2011). Social cognition as a mediator variable between neurocognition and functional outcome in schizophrenia: Empirical review and new results by structural equation modeling. *Schizophrenia Bulletin, 37*(suppl. 2), s41–s54.

Schwarz, N., & Clore, G. L. (2007). Feelings and phenomenal experience. In A. Kruglanski & E. T. Higgins (Eds.), *Social psychology: Handbook of basic principles* (2nd ed., pp. 385–407). New York: Guilford.

Sergi, M. J., & Green, M. F. (2002). Social perception and early visual processing in schizophrenia. *Schizophrenia Research, 59,* 233–241.

Sergi, M. J., Rassovsky, Y., Widmark, C., Reist, C., Erhart, S., Braff, D. L., . . . & Green, M. F. (2007). Social cognition in schizophrenia: Relationships with neurocognition and negative symptoms. *Schizophrenia Research, 90*(1–3), 316–324.

Van Overwalle, F. (2009). Social cognition and the brain: A meta-analysis. *Human Brain Mapping, 30*(3), 829–858.